IMPERATIVES OF CARE

HAWAI'I STUDIES ON KOREA

Imperatives of Care

Women and Medicine in Colonial Korea

SONJA M. KIM

University of Hawai'i Press, Honolulu
and
Center for Korean Studies, University of Hawai'i

Library of Congress Cataloging-in-Publication Data

Names: Kim, Sonja M., author.
Title: Imperatives of care : women and medicine in colonial Korea / by Sonja M. Kim.
Other titles: Hawai'i studies on Korea.
Description: Honolulu : University of Hawai'i Press : Center for Korean Studies, University of Hawai'i, [2019] | Series: Hawai'i studies on Korea | Includes bibliographical references and index.
Identifiers: LCCN 2018014809 | ISBN 9780824855451 (cloth ; alk. paper)
Subjects: LCSH: Women in medicine—Korea—History. | Women—Health and hygiene—Korea—History. | Reproductive health—Korea—History.
Classification: LCC R692 .K47 2019 | DDC 610.8209519—dc23
LC record available at https://lccn.loc.gov/2018014809

ISBN 978-0-8248-8840-4 (pbk.)

 The Center for Korean Studies was established in 1972 to coordinate and develop resources for the study of Korea at the University of Hawai'i. Reflecting the diversity of the academic disciplines represented by affiliated members of the university faculty, the Center seeks especially to promote interdisciplinary and intercultural studies. Hawai'i Studies on Korea, published jointly by the Center and the University of Hawai'i Press, offers a forum for research in the social sciences and humanities pertaining to Korea and its people.

Cover photo: "Salvation-for-all-women" Hospital (Poguyŏgwan), Seoul, 1907. Photograph courtesy of the United Methodist Church Archives, GCAH, Madison, New Jersey.

CONTENTS

ACKNOWLEDGMENTS

It has been said that writing a book is a labor of love. It is also a humbling experience, intensely challenging mentally, physically, and intellectually. I have been blessed to receive much support and inspiration over the years for which I am deeply grateful.

First, I would like to express my deepest gratitude to my professors while a graduate student at the University of California, Los Angeles (UCLA): John Duncan, George Dutton, Charlotte Furth, Benjamin Elman, Henry Em, Namhee Lee, Gi-Wook Shin, the late Miriam Silverberg, and Sharon Traweek. I also thank Kim Do-hyung, Jung Tae-hern, and the late Pang Kie-Chung for welcoming me in their graduate courses at Korea University and Yonsei University. Their classes, discussions, and examples fostered and continue to shape who I am as a scholar today.

I am also indebted to Yeo Inseok, Park Yunjae, and Sihn Kyuhwan for their continued collegiality and invitation to collaborative study and research at the Department of Medical History at Yonsei University. Conversations with Paul Cha, John Cheng, Hyaeweol Choi, Todd Henry, Kyung Moon Hwang, Jung Keun-Sik, Jennifer Jung-Kim, Michael Kim, Kim Ock-Joo, Kim Tae-Ho, Kwon Bodurae, Robert Ku, Seung-Ah Lee, Yoonkyung Lee, Lim Jongtae, Sung Deuk Oak, Jin-kyung Park, Youngju Ryu, Soyoung Suh, Stella Xu, and Theodore Jun Yoo provided valuable insight and directed me to new questions and sources. The book's development also benefited from my engagements with discussants, fellow panel members, and audiences at various venues I presented, including the Annual Meeting of the Association for Asian Studies, the Australian National University, Berkshire Conference on the History of Women, Cornell University, Hamilton College, Korea University,

University of Hong Kong, University of Illinois, Urbana-Champaign, University of Michigan, University of Toronto, and Yonsei University.

Special thanks are reserved for Su Yun Kim and Leighanne Yuh for their thoughtful reading, Kathy Ragsdale for her incisive editing, and two anonymous readers and my editor Stephanie Chun at the University of Hawai`i Press for their astute suggestions. I also thank my cohorts and classmates at UCLA whose friendship in and outside the classroom sustained me during and after graduate school. Colleagues at my home institution, the State University of New York at Binghamton, welcomed me in their programs, departments, and writing group as well as their homes and lives, furthering my growth as an academic, writer, and human being. My students with their passions and questions remind me daily why I teach and write.

This work was supported by the Core University Program for Korean Studies through the Ministry of Education of Republic of Korea and Korean Studies Promotion Service of the Academy of Korean Studies (AKS-2011-BAA-2103). Other institutions that made the book possible since its early stages include the Committee on Korean Studies of the Northeast Asia Council—Association for Asian Studies, Fulbright-Hays Program, Korea Foundation, UCLA, the Harpur College Dean's Office at Binghamton University, and the Fulbright US Scholar Program. I also thank the staff at the General Commission on Archives and History of the United Methodist Church, Presbyterian Historical Archives, Institute of the History of Christianity in Korea, Dong-Eun Medical Museum at Yonsei University College of Medicine, and the rare book collections of Drexel University, Ewha Womans University, Korea University, Seoul National University, UCLA, University of Toronto, and Yonsei University. My gracious hosts in Korea, the Institute of Korean Studies at Yonsei University and Kyujanggak Institute for Korean Studies at Seoul National University, provided me with the space, resources, and community that facilitated my research and writing.

Finally, I thank my relatives in Korea and in-laws in San Francisco for being my home away from home; my parents Myunghee and Kiljung Kim for their unfailing love, my sister Rosanne and my husband Jae for being my rocks; and Milena whose arrival forever shifted my view of history and motherhood. They have sustained me throughout this long journey, and it is to them I dedicate this book.

INTRODUCTION

In 1899, the vernacular newspaper *Cheguk sinmun* reported that a young woman, identified only as living in the neighborhood of Pukch'on, had approached Chi Sŏgyŏng, the principal of the newly opened Government Medical School, asking permission to matriculate.[1] He denied her appeal, informing her that although he found her intentions admirable, there were no provisions for females to study alongside male students. Undeterred, she petitioned the minister of education, an act the *Cheguk sinmun* praised as remarkable. According to the newspaper, the applicant initially hoped to attend the girls' school rumored soon to be established.[2] She reasoned, however, that as it remained unclear when that school would open and whether formal education would afford her as a woman (literally, "with a female body") the same opportunities as men, she instead should seek medical training, for it would provide her with "skills of use to the world" on a par with men.

The woman's request came during a dynamic period in Korea's history. Internal social strife, new treaty and international relations, and China's defeat by Japan in 1895, which signaled the end of the Sino-centric world order on which the Chosŏn (1392–1910) kingdom's polity was based, created a profound sense of crisis.[3] Concerned Korean leaders reconceptualized their understanding of "civilization" and accelerated reform efforts aimed at bolstering Chosŏn's sovereignty. The *Cheguk sinmun*'s praise for this woman incorporated her into an evolving modernist agenda. Her aspirations to acquire education in a newly founded institution and to procure medical expertise lay at the nexus of two key desires of Korean reformers: to improve the health of the population and thus the strength of the polity, and to provide women with skills to contribute to society.

1

What skills and what contributions were appropriate for women, however, were controversial issues in a society that, despite the efforts of reformers, remained highly ambivalent about the professionalization of women and even their work outside of conventional domestic prescriptions. The applicant from Pukch'ŏn's lack of confidence in the prospects for a new school for girls and her concern that, even if she were to graduate from that school, her abilities would be underappreciated, reveal continuing uncertainty about women's work and education. Although the Korean women's association Ch'anyanghoe (Promotion Society) received general support for its highly publicized 1898 petition to establish a girls' school, its efforts also stoked heated debate over the propriety of women's education. It was not just Chosŏn's gendered practices but also a noncommittal government that impeded the expansion of education for girls and women.[4] Before 1905, girls' schools, almost all established by foreign Protestant missionaries, had difficulty recruiting and retaining students. Even after a flurry of foundings of private girls' schools after Korea became a protectorate of Japan in 1905, the establishment of Hansŏng Girls' High School by the Korean state in 1908, and a primary education system established after Japan's colonization of Korea in 1910, education for women remained limited in its reach. Statistics compiled by the Government-General of Korea (GGK) show that as late as 1930, only about 6.6 percent of Korea's female population had any kind of primary education. The figure had risen to a mere 14.5 percent by 1937.[5]

Medical work, however, for various reasons proved an exception to the generally slow expansion of opportunities for women, albeit one that nonetheless suffered from the constraints of conservative biases. A 1909 editorial in the publication of the academic society Taehan Hŭnghakhoe urged that since it was impractical to eradicate traditions of spatial division between men and women, women should study in order to be able to practice medicine on women.[6] Indeed, it was partially in response to prescribed and gendered spatial divisions that the Chosŏn court implemented the *ŭinyŏ* or female medical worker system shortly after the founding of the kingdom and obliged the request of foreign Protestant missionaries in the 1880s for Korean women to assist them in their medical work.[7] Emerging priorities in public health and birthing practices around the turn of the twentieth century further legitimated roles for female medical workers as smallpox vaccinators and medical assistants as well as in obstetrics. Private and state nursing and midwifery programs were begun in the 1900s, and opportunities for women in these fields became even more prevalent after 1910. New routines in hospitals and clinical administration, moreover, necessitated the employment of trained nurses. In contrast to the Chosŏn dynasty, when *ŭinyŏ* were relegated to the lowest social status, the Japanese colonial period (1910–1945) witnessed the growth of medicine, midwifery, and nursing as prestigious, reputable, and potentially lucrative occupations for women.

Yet women in the early twentieth century still could not matriculate in medical school. Women who desired to become doctors had to choose alternate fields altogether such as midwifery or nursing, or resort to study abroad, usually in Japan, or privately, often under the tutelage of foreign missionaries. It was not until 1928, when the Korean Women's Medical Training Institute (*Chosŏn yŏja ŭihak kangsŭpso*, hereafter the Training Institute) began teaching its first class that women were able to attain systematically the sort of medical education to which the woman from Pukch'on had aspired decades earlier.[8]

The Training Institute graduated its first class of five in 1934. From its humble beginning, run initially by volunteer administrators and instructors who received no salary, it went on to earn accreditation by the GGK in 1938, raising its status to a specialized medical training college, the Keijō Women's Medical College (*Kyŏngsŏng yŏja ŭihak chŏnmun hakkyo*), thereby earning for its graduates licenses to practice medicine.[9] By the 1940s, the women's medical college was graduating over fifty students a year. Moreover, statistics show that while licensed Japanese nurses and midwives in Korea continued to outnumber their Korean counterparts throughout this period, the gap had significantly diminished by the 1940s. Medical education and professional work for women had become a permanent part of the Korean medical scene.

This book traces these dramatic changes in the role of women in health care, arguing for the centrality of gender politics in Korea's medical modernization from the late Chosŏn dynasty through Japanese colonial rule. Transforming visions of womanhood valorized motherhood and maternalism in ways different from those of the past, reinforcing the responsibility of women for care work. The reach of women's vigilance in protecting the health of others and themselves gradually extended beyond their homes to their communities and to the larger polity. These expanding duties gave rise to novel organizations of care in hospitals and the home, particularly as public health priorities in maternal and infant welfare privileged the reproductive health of the populace. The ensuing gendered practices shaped women's medical professionalization, health care activities, and experiences as patients and recipients of new medical knowledge in their varied roles as housewives, mothers, students, research subjects, and consumers. Women accordingly came to embody contradictions in the realm of health care and, more broadly, the practice of modern life that science and medicine promised.

A SHIFTING MEDICAL LANDSCAPE

Medicine, understood as the "science and art dealing with the maintenance of health and the prevention, alleviation, or cure of disease," has a history on the Korean peninsula of many centuries.[10] The Chosŏn court systematized a medical curriculum that derived its authority from a key text of the classical Chinese tradition, the *Inner Canon of the Yellow Emperor* (Ch. *Huangdi neijing*; K. *Hwangje naegyŏng*), access to which required a level of erudition available mainly to a small and educated male elite.[11] The court also established a medical bureaucracy that attended to public health administration (for example, the regulation of *materia medica*, managing epidemics, or providing famine relief) and the medical care of royal and elite families. Nevertheless, despite trends in the late Chosŏn period such as growth in the publication of medical texts and an expanding private medical sector with drug markets and itinerant healers, many forms of medical care were simply out of reach for the majority of the population. Medicinal ingredients to fulfill a physician's prescription were relatively expensive, and state medical institutions served primarily the capital-based population.[12]

What were available to the people at large were competing therapeutic methods and understandings of illness that contributed to a pluralistic medical terrain. Common treatments included medicine based on folk recipes, moxibustion and acupuncture, incantation, consultation with a blind fortune-teller, and shamanic rituals or the setting up of "idol-posts" at entrances to villages to expel illness-provoking evil

spirits.[13] Techniques of smallpox variolation through human inocula-
tion (*indubŏp*) had spread by the mid-nineteenth century.[14] Such folk
health practices, which drew from religious and popular beliefs, existed
alongside Confucian scholarly or elite health-seeking practices. In fact,
records indicate that many Koreans did not limit themselves to one system of medicine or healing tradition but drew on multiple resources in
the care of their bodies.[15]

It was not until the opening of treaty-specified ports to foreign trade
and settlements as well as new forms of diplomatic relations, starting with
the Japan-Korea Treaty of 1876 (also known as the Treaty of Kanghwa),
that Chosŏn reformers became significantly interested in and familiar
with what Ruth Rogaski argues is the major point of divergence between
the Western European and Sino-classical medical spheres: Western
forms of organization with respect to medical services and public sanitation including sewage, a safe water supply, and contagious disease control.[16] Such practices became framed by Chosŏn reformers as integral
to efforts in self-strengthening and "civilizing" along new rubrics in a
rapidly changing world. In this they were inspired in particular by the
developing concept of *wisaeng* (Ch. *weisheng*; J. *eisei*) that Rogaski translates as "hygienic modernity" and that "link the government, the police,
the laboratory, and the people in one encompassing project of national
health."[17] Discussions on health and medical reforms emerged in memo-
rials to the throne, reports from observation missions, personal writings,
and in the nascent print media.[18] Guided by the political framework of
"Eastern Way, Western Techniques" (*Tongdo sŏgi*) with its highly selective adoption of new knowledge, technologies (particularly those related
to the military, transportation, communication, and electricity), economic tools, and diplomatic and administrative protocols based on foreign models, the Chosŏn state initiated modest reforms in public health
such as smallpox vaccination and quarantines on a limited scale.[19] It also
appointed American Protestant missionary Horace Allen, the physician
to the U.S. legation who had won the favor of the court with his treatment
of officials and of Queen Min's nephew, Min Yong'ik, in the aftermath
of the 1884 Kapsin Coup, as attendant physician of a new royal hospital
Chejungwŏn that treated patients based on Western techniques.[20]

In the aftermath of the Sino-Japanese War (1894–1895), Korean
reformers' "decentering China" agenda drew yet further on Japanese and

Western institutional models and material goods to address the social and political ills blamed for the widespread and nearly kingdom-toppling popular rebellions, and to fortify Korea against foreign encroachment.[21] In particular, as King Kojong promulgated his polity as the Great Han Empire (*Taehan cheguk*, hereafter, the Taehan state) and declared himself emperor in 1897, reformers redefined the nature of the state, its ruler, and its relations with not only foreign powers but also its own people, thereby altering visions for the responsibilities, duties, expectations, rights, and privileges of both the ruler and the population.[22] This became evident in the realm of public health as reformers repackaged the moral values of the monarch's benevolence displayed in the care of his subjects' welfare and the subjects' loyalty to their ruler as, respectively, the state's obligation to protect the health of the populace through sanitary and medical regulations, institutions, and projects and the individual's civic responsibility to discipline personal bodily and health practices. Linking the health of individuals outward organically with the household, local community, state, and later empire, formed the rationale for emerging public health initiatives and intensified forms of interventions such as compulsory quarantines and regulations on personal comportment administered by a Bureau of Hygiene established in 1894 and enforced by a new sanitary police system aimed at supporting the enforcement of sanitary regulations.[23]

Administrators developed a growing interest in biomedicine and increasingly promoted new sanitary practices with which the populace was to identify. This emulation was reflected in the Taehan state's new public health and medical administration, such as the guidelines issued for the prevention of cholera and reorganization of the Bureau of Hygiene—now expanded to regulate medical professions, hospitals, and sales of medicines in addition to managing the control of diseases.[24] Graduates of the Training School for Vaccinators served as vaccination officials, appointed to perform smallpox vaccinations in the capital and provincial areas.[25] The state started a government medical school in 1899 that included biomedicine in its curriculum and hired physicians trained in both Western and Korean traditions to serve in the newly established government hospital Kwangjewŏn ("House of Extended Deliverance") and prisons.[26] Licensing regulations promulgated in 1900 to standardize medical and pharmaceutical professions were inspired by Japanese and Western models but, according to Soyoung Suh's analysis, defined a physician as one versed in Sino-classical medical cosmologies, thereby demonstrating that "although [reformers] understood the significance of implementing biomedicine in Korea, a systematic plan for replacing traditional medicine with biomedicine was hardly on their minds."[27]

In addition, hospitals and physicians treating patients in accordance with biomedicine and Western practices increasingly began to appear on the Korean landscape. Japanese settlements conducted sanitation projects and employed military surgeons in hospitals established in the treaty-port areas of Pusan (1877) and Wŏnsan (1880), as well as the capital Seoul (1883). While these hospitals treated primarily the Japanese resident population, they also provided free medical treatment to Korean natives in an attempt, as argued by Pak Yunjae, to mollify anti-Japanese sentiment and convey a sense of Japanese superiority among the Korean populace.[28] Other Japanese physicians seeking new opportunities migrated to Korea and opened private practices. The Japanese medical organization Dōjinkai (K. *Tonginhoe*, "the Universal Benevolence Organization") formed in 1902 with the goal of sending physicians and pharmacists abroad to areas of Japan's imperialist ambitions, began to dispatch Japanese physicians to Korea in 1904 with the outbreak of the Russo-Japanese War.[29] These physicians worked with local hygiene administrations and established hospitals near major rail centers, some of which later became incorporated into the public charity-provincial hospital system run by the Japanese colonial administration.[30]

Moreover, despite the Chosŏn court's explicit ban on Christian evangelism, Horace Allen and Chejungwŏn paved the way for the entry of foreign Protestant missionaries whose medical and educational work were tolerated. Their activities introduced Western medical practices to larger segments of the Korean population, especially as mission boards appointed medical missionaries to nearly all stations in the interior and transformed Chejungwŏn (renamed Severance Hospital in 1904) into a major institution of medical care and education after the Chosŏn court relinquished control of its administration in 1894.[31] While missionaries did not expend much energy on public health administration, except in support of the state's disease control efforts in, for example, quarantines and isolation hospitals in times of major epidemics, they valued hygienic habits perceived as integral to leading a Christian life and thus provided simple instructions on personal health from the pulpit, through the schools they operated, and in the Christian literature they published.[32]

When Korea became a protectorate of Japan in 1905 after the Russo-Japanese War, the Japanese Resident-General of Korea (hereafter RG) increasingly took control of the Taehan state's public health and medical administration, with enforcement provided by an enhanced Sanitary Police aided by police physicians. This shifted after annexation with the establishment of the public physician (*kongŭi*) system in 1914, which employed physicians to assist in public health work, work in public dispensaries, and supplement the work of police physicians, particularly in outlying areas that lacked a charity hospital.[33] In 1907, the RG replaced the former government hospital Kwangjewŏn, its affiliated medical school, and the Red Cross Hospital with a new hospital, the Taehan Hospital (*Taehan ŭiwŏn*), designed to display Japan's prowess in modern science and medicine. It was as formidable in its appearance as it was in its organization. Consisting of departments of internal medicine, surgery, ophthalmology, obstetrics-gynecology, otolaryngology, pediatrics, dermatology, and dentistry, with staff members including physicians, teachers, pharmacists, translators, and technicians, the Taehan Hospital was intended to offer specialized advanced treatment, rather than act as a relief hospital in the manner that Kwangjewŏn had, although it did continue to treat indigent Korean patients on a limited scale.[34] Moreover, all public health administrative work (including contagious disease management, medical licensing and education, and hospital administration) was transferred to Taehan Hospital, divesting the Taehan state completely of jurisdiction over public health and medicine. And with promulgation of new licensing requirements for medical professions within a few years after annexation, the colonial state tightened control over the medical activities of foreign missionaries and affirmed biomedicine as the organizing principle of the developing medical system in colonial Korea.[35] It is this context in which events addressed in this book unfolded.

REPRODUCTION AS AN
ORGANIZING PRINCIPLE

Overhaul of the Taehan state's public health and medical infrastructure was framed by the logic of achieving healthier bodies, initially to strengthen the Taehan position in the competition for survival among nations, later to serve Japanese imperialist ambitions after 1905. At the same time, these goals promoted a maternalist agenda that supported women's public participation superficially in their biological and social roles as mothers. Women's political and cultural contributions were no longer to be restricted to the maintenance of familial harmony or the faithful observance of particular rites or rituals, but now, most importantly, included the birthing and raising of the future generation. This priority focused discussions of women's status on their sexuality and physical bodies.[36] It was primarily through their reproductive activities as mothers that women were to be integrated into modern Korean society.

Korean reformers who articulated these maternalist ideals echoed trends in other parts of the world around this period, though without opening a path to the sorts of activism to which maternalism led elsewhere. In Western Europe and the United States, notions that "exalted women's capacity to mother and extended to society as a whole the values of care, nurturance, and morality" allowed women to mobilize and organize for social reform, particularly in areas relating to the welfare of women and children.[37] Although the breadth and goals of maternalist policies largely were designed by male officials and foreign Protestant medical missionaries, it was educated women who benefited from the opportunities afforded by those policies and who, necessarily, were the ones to implement them. Attempts, for example, to regulate and train personnel in new childbirth practices were part of this agenda, and intersected with the general standardization and professionalization of medical work. The period witnessed processes that medicalized childbirth by differentiating between normal and abnormal deliveries but, because there was not yet a shift in the spatial location of childbirth from the home to the hospital, a need for medical midwives emerged specifically to attend to births in women's homes. In such fashion, new possibilities opened for women to work professionally in medicine, midwifery, and nursing.

Moreover, instructions for women on proper health practices were not limited to those seeking a health career but were conducted through the Domestic Sciences curriculum in girls' schools and public health programs such as informational campaigns and fairs, infant welfare clinics, and home visits. These activities were guided by the perception of women as guardians of their family's health and thus focused on the techniques and hygienic principles women were to apply in their care of children and household tasks such as cooking, cleaning, and even sewing. In addition, women were to learn to *know* their bodies in new ways.[38] Debates on sex education and birth control, descriptions of women's physiological ailments, and patent medical advertisements in print media reveal the ways that at least literate women were to come to know and be responsible for their reproductive health.

A gendered analysis of medical history offers further insights into how medicine produced, and in turn was produced by, gendered expectations. The new service of care offered in hospitals, for example, depended on the nursing profession, which became gendered female at this time. Disproportionate attention to women's reproductive system and function shaped the medical literature and services made available. Ironically, it sustained rather than ending or replacing older medical traditions usually targeted for eradication or castigation by a modernist medical agenda. Moreover, despite being the persons directly affected by maternal practices, women found their voices and women-centered concerns overshadowed by pronatalist desires and men who shaped policies and services relating to maternal and child welfare. Yet these very concerns, while increasing forms of medical intervention and surveillance by colonial authorities and health institutions, could also provide a basis for advocacy for women's health concerns, particularly when they related to the enhancement of women's fertility.

Imperatives of Care addresses the social, cultural, political, and medical implications that emerged from transforming notions of womanhood and public health practices in the context of Korean nationalism, Japanese imperialism, and Christian mission evangelism in the late nineteenth and early twentieth centuries. As such, it is about the politics of health care, the processes involved in defining matters of and pursuits related to health. It is also about reproductive politics, the struggle over making decisions in matters of pregnancy, childbirth, and child-rearing.[39] To consider these issues, this book focuses on the experiences of women in three general areas of inquiry: health and female education, professionalization of female medical workers, and women's and infants' health care and therapeutics.

The first chapter, "Sanitizing Women and the Domestic Sciences," examines the early twentieth-century production of a new cluster of academic subjects in female education. This cluster included instruction in physiology, nursing, "household matters (*kasa*)," and household management that sought to apply the medical, scientific, and technological practices of the period to the performance of women's tasks within the home. The Domestic Sciences emerged initially in new mission schools for girls on an inconsistent basis depending on the availability of teachers, but was introduced to students informally through their performance of daily routines stipulated by dormitory regulations. It became more defined as educators and Korean male reformers published textbooks and formalized a household-related curriculum in girls' schools, both public and private, drawing upon Meiji Japanese models of female education and American home economics. Analyzing this curriculum in contrast to the curriculum presented by late Chosŏn period moral primers and handbooks for women, this chapter asserts that the new forms of female education endeavored to cultivate a particular type of *kungmin* or "citizen-subject" of the state that demanded of a woman the duty of caring for the health of her family and her maternal body without necessarily ensuring her access to rights or opportunities. Mission schools shared similar visions of domesticity that stressed connections to women's larger communities. The privileging of women's care-providing roles allowed schools to imagine sciences broadly in the training of female students for their future roles and encouraged female students' higher education in the sciences and health fields.

The following chapter, "From the *Ŭinyŏ* to the *Yŏ'ŭi*: The Female Physician," traces the emergence of medicine as a legitimate profession for women as it evolved from new legal and institutional infrastructures in public health and medical systems implemented initially by the Taehan state and foreign Protestant missionaries and administered later by the GGK. The chapter also provides a brief overview of medical care in the Chosŏn period as it transitioned during the colonial period to modern public health and medical institutions. The participation of women in medicine in the early twentieth century is best understood when situated in the context of Korean modernist desires, the biopolitics of the Japanese colonial state, foreign missionary visions for female education and medicine, and professionalization of medical personnel in general. The complex synergy among new meanings attached to women's reproduction, medical work, and "motherly" or maternal nature shaped the education and professional experiences of newly trained female medical workers.

Chapter three, "The Heavenly Task of Nursing," examines the participation of missionaries in the professionalization of nursing and midwifery, particularly through their engagements in infant welfare programs to combat the infant mortality that presented a threat to the social fabric and moral order of colonial Korea. Filling a vacuum they perceived in the Japanese colonial public health administration, mission infant welfare programs expanded in the context of what Kim Hyegyŏng calls the "medicalization of the family" in 1920s and 1930s print media, the GGK's health and lifestyle campaigns to "improve daily life" and "love and protect the child," the growth of pediatrics and psychology as legitimate medical specialties, and shifting conceptualizations of children and the home.[40] These programs, though limited in scope and reach, did promote the training of Korean women in midwifery and public health nursing and developed Korean female leadership in professional medical, public health, and social services.

The focus on reproduction in women's medicine is reflected in the final chapter, "Negotiating Gynecology: Constant Imperatives, Evolving Options." It explores the kinds of medical activities directed at women's bodies and the related knowledge and goods produced for and consumed by women to assess concerns held in regard to women's health, the perception and treatment of the female body, and the ways individual women sought to intervene in those practices. The nebulous disease category *puinbyŏng* ("women's disease") offers a fascinating example of the ways modern practices and knowledge of the body and medicine re-appropriated older traditions. Associated with a broad array of practices ranging from fertility treatment, postpartum care, birth control, and general health care, the developing specialty of gynecology privileged the reproductive health of the populace over other health concerns, determined by the logic of a tradition that was difficult to break. Nevertheless, seizing the knowledge and services made available to them empowered women to take measures to secure healthier and more fulfilling lives.

Throughout the book, I employ the McCune-Reischauer romanization for Korean terms and names, indicating in parentheses the preferred spelling when supplied. Chinese is rendered in Pinyin and Japanese in Hepburn respectively. I write well-known terms like "Seoul" in their conventional spelling. When citing directly from historical sources, I use the transliteration as written in the original. Surnames appear first without the comma for historical figures and authors in East Asia. Translations are mine unless otherwise indicated.

CHAPTER 1

Sanitizing Women and the Domestic Sciences

Spurred by a sense of crisis as foreign powers battled to expand their spheres of influence on the peninsula after China's defeat by Japan in 1895, Koreans sought means to bolster Chosŏn's sovereignty. In the course of this, they redefined their understanding of "civilization" and constructed new definitions for what it meant to be a member of Chosŏn, Taehan, and the Korean nation (*minjok*).[1] Korean reformers accelerated their efforts to change international relations, the government bureaucracy, education, and the social order, inspired by concepts ranging from the more radical "Civilization and Enlightenment" (*munmyŏng kaehwa*) to the more selective "Maintain Old Foundations, Add the New" (*kubon sinch'am*).[2] One area of central concern was the status of women, with a concomitant focus on the domestic sphere and its related institutions (household, family, marriage) and practices (housework, cottage industries, child-rearing, etc.). That the most intimate human relations among family members drew the attention of reformers was not a new phenomenon. Based on Confucian worldviews that cosmically linked the domestic sphere not only to the rise and fall of the dynasty but also to a universal harmony of "all under heaven," the Chosŏn court targeted kinship practices, promoted Confucian values of filiality and wifely chastity, and prescribed spatial and symbolic divisions in the home based on sex.[3] Late nineteenth- and early twentieth-century reform advocates similarly grounded the fortunes of the larger collective on the family unit, in which the roles of women were critical.

Among these reformers was Yu Kilchun, who radically reinterpreted ideals for the treatment and education of women in his magnum opus *Sŏyu kyŏnmun* (Observations on a journey to the West, 1895).[4] While he framed his work as an impartial record, his intent was quite plain. The West, he reported, no longer used the gendered divisions between inner and outer spheres so prevalent in Chosŏn society and thought. He asserted, furthermore, that education was what provided humanity to a woman: "An uneducated woman is unable to do what she should do as a human being. . . . Women are different from men, but are they not also human beings?" Here, Yu voiced an early and forceful call for the formal schooling of women. While female education, particularly among the elite, had been important to families and the state throughout the Chosŏn dynasty, it was conducted within the domicile largely through moral primers and family instruction on household tasks.[5] Yu, however, explained that in the West people had "establish[ed] various means to educate women beginning in childhood." Moreover, while women "have the primary responsibility for educating children," they also assume male duties abandoned at times of war, for example, or make "contributions to society as important as those made by men." Thus, women must learn matters related to not only "cloth-ing, liquor, or food," but also subjects that would enable them to "be con-versant in the principles of all worldly affairs and even to know the niceties of such things as music and arithmetic." In other words, education for women was to be reconceived on new grounds. Not only the content but also the purpose and application of female education needed to change.

Female education became a significant component in the transfor-mation of the domestic sphere at the turn of the twentieth century. Not only did schools for girls challenge earlier spatial divisions that justified their exclusion from formal education and work in areas convention-ally rendered male, but an evolving female curriculum also promoted a concept of womanhood that oriented them toward roles in the domestic realm in ways qualitatively different from previous times. The casting of women as guardians of the health of their families, especially in their capacities as mothers, intersected with general efforts to improve the health of the population. On the one hand, this reflected the medical reality of rampant and devastating epidemics in a society with limited awareness and application of germ theory, inadequate public sanita-tion services, weak medical infrastructure, and the absence of effective therapeutics. On the other, it revealed gendered roles women were now expected to perform as part of general efforts to mobilize the population for state, Christian, and nation-building goals. These agendas shaped curriculums including the sciences in women's formal schooling and women's place in the nascent public health and medical system.

Accordingly, a new cluster of academic subjects I refer to as the Domestic Sciences emerged in the female-gendered curriculum at the turn of the twentieth century. I use Domestic Sciences in the plural and capitalized to differentiate it from the singular "domestic science" commonly used interchangeably with "home economics" and to high-light the flexibility and permeability of household-related subjects. This was not a set program of study with a clearly defined syllabus or agenda. Rather, the Domestic Sciences was an amalgam of some-times disparate, occasionally conflicting, yet overall interconnected subjects that varied depending on the time period, level of education (primary, middle, secondary, vocational, specialized), and particular school. While it centered primarily on the subject of home econom-ics as it evolved in this period, denoted initially by the Meiji Japanese neologism *kajŏnghak* (J. *kaseigaku*, literally "the study of household management") and later in the colonial period by *kasa* (J. *kaji*, vari-ably translated as "household matters," "housekeeping," or "domestic affairs"), Domestic Sciences as used here included other subjects like *chaebong* (sewing or tailoring), *suye* (manual arts or handicraft), and various subcategories of the natural sciences such as *wisaeng* (hygiene) and *saengnihak* (physiology).

This chapter compares and contrasts the Domestic Sciences curric-ulum against earlier Chosŏn period primers and the textbooks of other curricular subjects to demonstrate both the overlap and shift in the con-cept of household management in general and female education in par-ticular. The Domestic Sciences as it unfolded in schools and popular media idealized the home, instructed its management, and informed what it meant to be a modern woman of the era. The privileging of wom-en's care-providing roles placed directives on hygiene and sanitation at the forefront of their education, shaping the kinds of scientific and tech-nical education female students began to receive. Nevertheless, finding themselves relegated to the new domestic realm, women discovered that the promises of the modern eluded them despite the articulation of their importance to their families and by extension their communities, the state, and, eventually, the Japanese empire.

FROM THE INNER QUARTERS
TO THE CLASSROOM

The September 1898 "A Petition for a Women's School" signed by members of the women-organized Ch'anyanghoe (Promotion Society) was reprinted and discussed in various newspapers of the time.[6] Addressed to the king, it promoted the cause of women's formal education, calling specifically for state attention to women's schools. While the reorganized Board of Education and private school administrators focused their attentions on the creation of new schools and a curriculum for boys, as of 1898 there was only a handful of schools for girls, established primarily by foreign Protestant missionaries, starting with Ewha Girls' School in 1886.[7] Couched in the "Civilization and Enlightenment" language of its times, Ch'anyanghoe's plea, like that of Yu Kilchun, firmly framed the formal education of women within the larger discourse of nation building while appealing to Confucian sensibilities. The founders asserted that their activities stemmed from their "commitment, loyalty, and devotion" to the king, for His Majesty had urged "realizing the task of independence" by establishing public schools.[8] The United States and countries in Europe "reached enlightenment and progress by establishing schools for women." Thus, the establishment of a women's school in Chosŏn would serve "the purpose of making this country prosperous from the women's quarters." When the state did not fulfill its initial commitment to start a government girls' school, Ch'anyanghoe established the private Sunsŏng Girls' School later that year.

A decade later the state followed suit with the founding of the Hansŏng Girls' High School in 1908.[9] This was an epochal step, for throughout the Chosŏn dynasty formal education was out of reach for the majority of the population, especially women, in that schools were closely associated with preparations for the civil service examination system, the prerogative of *yangban* men and the means for official appointment that conferred elite status in Chosŏn society.[10] As such, qualified young boys who aspired to enter officialdom studied privately or at local schools, moving through official channels that culminated with the Royal Confucian Academy (*Sŏnggyungwan*) at the capital. The Chosŏn state also offered instruction to royal family members as well as the lower-status *chungin*, bureaucrat-technicians such as interpreters.

Except for female workers of the state like *kisaeng* entertainers or *ŭinyŏ* medical workers, women did not have access to formal education.

While schooling may have been limited, education in general was an integral and significant part of the Chosŏn polity, woven into the moral fabric of the social order. Learning was a task required of all people, not as a means of individual fulfillment but as self-cultivation with implications for one's household and, by extension, one's country and the cosmos. Education thus served several purposes. On the one hand, it offered men training in preparation for examinations and in specialized skills for the performance of assigned tasks. On the other hand, education allowed individuals to activate their moral capacities and maintain proper human social relations. The Chosŏn court sponsored publications of Confucian canonic literature in the vernacular script in order to teach women and commoners their prescribed roles in the neo-Confucian social order that the state sought to institute.[11]

The education of women, particularly elite women, in the Chosŏn period must be considered in this light. The transformative neo-Confucian engineering implemented by the Chosŏn court at the beginning of the dynasty legislated kinship practices along strict patriarchal and patrilineal principles, which radically differed from the previous dynasty. This rearranged the roles, status, and responsibilities of women that had to be learned.[12] The complementary yet restrictive delineation between inner and outer spheres, women's full incorporation into their husbands' descent group upon marriage, and the ranking of wives placed women firmly within the domestic realm, their status and comportment having grave consequences for their husbands' lineage and sons' future prospects.[13] The link forged between the regulation of one's household and the kingdom meant that how a woman behaved in her husband's home affected the moral order of the cosmos. The proper performance of women's roles then was to be produced correctively through punitive measures and indirectly through education.[14]

Relegated rhetorically to the inner sphere and spatially to the household quarters, women from a young age received their education in their natal and husbands' homes. A separate genre of moral handbooks for this purpose proliferated, particularly in the latter half of the dynasty. Such texts included those commissioned by the state as well as those written for private use by family members.[15] Other didactic means included board games, lyric poem-songs that circulated among women in a household (*naebang* or *kyubang kasa*), and extra-literary forms such as shamanic songs and *p'ansori*, a popular oral narrative and performing art form in late Chosŏn.[16]

Instructive texts for women during the Chosŏn period focused over-whelmingly on "womanly virtues" (*pudŏk*). While largely exhorted to follow the Confucian cardinal human principles of filiality (*hyo*) and loyalty (*ch'ung*) also expected of men, elite women were to orient these principles primarily toward their husband's affines. In other words, the role prioritized for them was that of daughter-in-law and not necessarily mother. This perhaps accounts for why a woman's inability to conceive a son as grounds for divorce was overridden by considerations of her contributions to her husband's family, such as improving its economic situation or performing mourning rites for parents-in-law.[17] Women were to maintain harmonious relations among household members, uphold filial duties toward their parents-in-law, avoid jealousy and tension with other daughters-in-law in the household, and discipline servants with a firm yet compassionate hand. Doing so would ensure proper order in their husbands' household and lineage.

In addition to moral handbooks, practical guidebooks circulated among women. These focused on specific tasks women performed on behalf of their husbands' households. For example, the expectation to honor and receive guests following appropriate etiquette or protocols fell primarily on women, who had to know how to prepare and serve various liquors/wines and food. Much attention was also placed on food and other preparations women performed for *chesa*, the ancestral rites framed in this period as the central pillar in maintaining the lineage. This is exemplified by one of the more well-known encyclopedic guidebooks for women, *Kyuhap ch'ongsŏ*, compiled in 1809 by Madam Yi (1759–1824) of Pinghŏgak to circulate privately for reference and for the education of women in the household. The text did not focus on the moral qualities a woman was to possess to the extent of other female primers but instead provided detailed instructions on household-related tasks women generally performed in their roles as daughters-in-law such as how to ferment wine, prepare certain dishes, clean brassware and cooking utensils properly, and administer emergency first aid on simple wounds and injuries like snakebites.[18]

Instructions on child-rearing, however, were relatively scarce in both moral primers and practical handbooks. While *Kyuhap ch'ongsŏ* did include a short section on care during pregnancy, more information on this topic would have been found in medical-related tracts, such as the opus *Tongŭi pogam* (Precious mirror of Eastern medicine, 1613) or vernacular translations of obstetrics and pediatric texts, which were not necessarily gendered female.[19] Information in these texts ranged from an explanation of human life in Confucian cosmological terms and correlated techniques to conceive, obstetric-related information such as types of childbirth positions and how to dispose of the placenta, and prescriptions for pregnancy- and postpartum-related ailments such as infertility, morning sickness, edema, and low breast-milk production. That knowledge of proper conception, gestation, and delivery of a male child was desired and circulated among women by the late Chosŏn period is suggested by the private text *T'aegyo singi*, which echoed some of the information provided in medical texts such as how to change the sex of the fetus from female to male, foods prohibited during pregnancy, and places to avoid on specific months or days to prevent miscarriage.[20]

When the topic of the biological mother–child relationship itself arose, it was usually in the form of moral exhortations such as the rules by which women were to abide in their relationships with their children. For example, women were expected to raise stepchildren or children from their husband's earlier marriage(s).[21] Other instructions included those related to a parturient woman's emotions and conduct, argued to leave an imprint on the moral character and physicality of her unborn child. *Naehun*, a moral primer for women attributed to Queen Sohye (1437–1504), exhorted women to maintain moral fortitude during pregnancy and child-rearing. It also coached women to encourage children to use their right hands (become right-handed), the age children should start reading, and character traits they were to instill in their children. These skills relate to the proper calligraphy, literacy, and comportment required in Confucian self-cultivation and education.[22] Another text, *Kyenyŏsŏ*, written by the scholar Song Siyŏl (1607–1689) for his daughter, merely stressed that mothers were to teach morals to their children for their children's behavior would reflect back on them. Nevertheless, while women may have been concerned with conceiving and bearing healthy sons, it was not the case that child-rearing itself was a task solely relegated to women. One of the few records on child-rearing we have extant from the Chosŏn period is the *Yangarok* (Records of raising a child, Yi Mungŏn, 1494–1567), a detailed record kept by a male literatus of the upbringing, education, and medical care of his only grandson.

Moreover, Chosŏn period texts do not suggest that the responsibility and daily tasks related to the management of households lay with women. The term *kajŏng* (家政; J. *kasei*; literally "governing the household") held different resonance in this period than it did as part of the later configuration *kajŏnghak* that was used to indicate a newly conceived female curriculum in home economics around the turn of the twentieth century. *Kajŏng* in the eighteenth century was the title of a volume in the agricultural manual *Chŭngbo sannim kyŏngje* as well as the title of a single autonomous tract with similar content.[23] The domestic site referenced in these texts included the physical compound of the household, its attached lands and animals, and people associated whether by blood, marriage relations, or service (servants and slaves). The household (*ka*) was not merely the building in which family members resided and had their material needs met. It was also the site of production and household income. Its management thus included the technical crafts of weaving and sericulture as well as the proper distribution of the household finances for rituals and inheritance. What stands out in the volume *Kajŏng* of the *Chŭngbo sannim kyŏngje* is its striking moral tone, which resonates with the virtues present in female primers. The guiding principle in the management of the *ka* was the Confucian tenet *susin chega* ("regulate one's body in order to regulate one's household"), stipulating how one was to behave, eat, read, speak, and conduct rites. Here, too, the proper management of the household was premised on harmonious relations among household members: parents, parents-in-law, spouses, siblings, servants, relatives, neighbors. It also stipulated the moral education of one's children, including young daughters, as part of cultivating proper moral values in familial relations. The *ka* was thus a site of ethical human relations with cosmic ramifications.

Accordingly, the individual mainly accountable for household management was not a woman but the male household head. The fact that these texts were written in classical Chinese also attests to a likely landed educated male elite readership and authorship.[24] Women may have performed some of the tasks that contributed to the operations of a household but the main targets of *kajŏng* instructions were men. Responsibility for the proper (or improper) management of the household ultimately resided with men. This was also reflected in law as men would also be punished for failing to manage their wives in cases when their wives were convicted of murder or other acts of violence.[25] Assisting them in maintaining harmonious relations in the household were their daughters-in-law and wives. A strict gendered delineation between a male outer or public sphere of state politics-work and female inner or private sphere in the domicile did not exist in Chosŏn Korea.

Although the "Civilization and Enlightenment" agenda of the late Chosŏn period denigrated many practices of the past, one critical principle that persisted and was interwoven into the transforming polity was the classical association between the regulation of one's household and the kingdom soon-to-be nation and later empire. In this framework, reformers reconsidered the household and the women who operated within it. How women were to serve the changing needs in Chosŏn while assuming the primary position in the domestic sphere and the role of education in preparing them for their future tasks continued to be contested as formal schooling for girls began to take root.

THE GENDERED CONTOURS
OF CIVIC EDUCATION

Education, whether through schools or other institutions, public lectures and campaigns, print and other forms of media, standardized curriculums, or licensing and other qualifying examination systems, has often been understood in modern states to be not only a way to cultivate specific knowledge and skills but also an effective means of instilling in a targeted population perspectives and orientations that encourage desired behaviors and attitudes. The challenges posed by the new economic and diplomatic arrangements that came with Korea's opening in 1876 motivated some to establish Western-inspired schools that incorporated a new curriculum. Not surprisingly, some of the first schools of "new learning" were opened in the treaty ports of Wŏnsan (1883),

Pusan (1895), and Inch'ŏn (1900) by local residents who found novel subjects such as world geography, foreign languages, and international law useful in their daily lives as they engaged and competed with foreign traders.[26] Following the self-strengthening model of "Wealthy Country, Strong Army" (*puguk kangbyŏng*) in the 1880s, the state established its first government schools based on Western models by employing foreign instructors to train future officials in the English language, military techniques, and agricultural technology.[27] Other new-style schools for Koreans launched in the last decades before the nineteenth century included those established by Japanese settlers and Christian schools founded by foreign Protestant missionaries.[28]

The charged political atmosphere after China's defeat in the Sino-Japanese War stimulated increasing acceptance among Koreans of the "new learning" now seen as indispensable to Korea's civilizing agenda. While some of the 1894–1896 reforms implemented by the Kabo council supported by the Japanese presence in Seoul were later revoked or not enforced, educational reforms such as the abolishment of the civil service examinations that had served as the means of selecting officials, the establishment of the Office for Educational Affairs (Hangmu Amun, later renamed Ministry of Education), the expansion of public schools based on Japanese and Western models, and publication of government textbooks became permanent features. New educational policies and the activities they spurred reveal not only that the meaning of new learning had begun to take hold but also that the relationship between the monarch and his people was changing. The populace referred to as *kungmin*, *paeksŏng*, *inmin*, or just simply *min* in official documents and popular print media at the turn of the twentieth century were variously imagined as a community of persons, subjects of the monarch/emperor, citizens, the citizenry, or the people. Regardless of nomenclature, individuals began to experience the increasing reach of the state's efforts to redirect its relationship with them. The duties, obligations, and roles the state and the people were expected to perform for each other were articulated in the evolving government education system.

It is in this sense that Kyung Moon Hwang describes state efforts in public schooling in Korea after 1895, and the discursive terrain created in response, as "citizenship education." While using terms such as "citizenship" with their association with a liberal tradition in non-Asian contexts remains a topic of debate in Korean historiography, Hwang makes the case that textbooks, curriculums, and policies related to government schools reveal not only the kinds of knowledge and skills people were expected to gain to meet the challenges of the modern world, but also the visions of state authority and a collective social order that the state desired to ingrain in the people.[29] Accordingly, education was about the making of new citizens; Hwang translates *kungmin* to mean people who constitute the country and thus are subject to the authority of the state.[30] To be sure, the state's prioritization of the people's duties, obligations, and allegiance sometimes conflicted with other conceptions of what it meant to be a citizen.

The new educational system as initially presented by King Kojong in his 1895 educational decree (*Kyoyuk ipkuk chosŏ*; literally "Proclamation for Education as the Means to Establish the State"), posited the new learning as helping the people perform critical roles in the very preservation of Chosŏn ("If the people are not educated, it is difficult for the country to have strength . . . education is the foundation for preserving the country").[31] Stating that he is carrying on the Confucian imperatives of *kyohwa* ("edifying" or "civilizing") and benevolence that formed the basis of the kingdom's legitimacy for the past five-hundred-plus years as practiced by his predecessors, Kojong ordered his subjects, both officials and the common people within his realm, to pursue the new learning and heed his words as it was only they who were able to confront the weakness of Chosŏn, block insults from other countries, and perfect state politics. The "wealth and strength" of the country depended on their moral character, physical strength, and wisdom, which were to be cultivated through the new schools and directed toward reviving the country. This was pivotal because, at least on paper, the elite and commoners were both considered subject to the same education and schools, suggesting an unprecedented type of social parity.

Moreover, the people were obliged to express patriotism (*ch'ungae*, "loyalty and love") in their service toward the welfare of the larger collective and greater good. These lessons were most explicit in the ethics *susin* curriculum (morals or "self-cultivation"), perhaps the most important academic course in the primary and higher grades, a point reiterated in the 1906 Edict on Common Schools.[32] The teaching of ethics in schools was not unique to Korea, and educators and the state when preparing textbooks for publication drew upon models from other countries such as Japan and the United States.[33] In fact, the interweaving of existing practices in Confucian statecraft and self-cultivation in the evolving state- and nation-building agenda was common in both Japanese and Chinese textbooks of this period. While the first Chosŏn government–published textbook, *Kungmin sohak tokpon* (People's Elementary Reader, 1895), focused the majority of its chapters on new curriculums such as geography, history, natural sciences, and international law, it also asserted a Chosŏn-centered position in moralistic terms legible to students familiar with Confucian classical education. The "loyalty, filial piety, and obedience" of heroes drawn from past Korean kingdoms were to inspire students' future contributions to the welfare of the country.[34] These ideas circulated and dominated the "Civilization and Enlightenment" discourse on education. Missionaries likewise stressed character building in their schools, although with a Christian bent. Students were encouraged to contribute their talents and learning to their larger communities as Christians or in ways befitting a Christian life, and in this sense received a type of civic education that, even though it was not designed to do so, supported or overlapped with state objectives.[35]

After Korea became a protectorate of Japan following its victory in the Russo-Japanese War (1904–1905), the Resident-General (RG) took increasing control over Korea's foreign and domestic affairs.[36] It replaced officials in the Ministry of Education, instituted a new public school system with primary schools—renamed common schools—taught by Japanese teachers, and passed regulations on private schools and textbook publication. While the view that the function of public education was to discipline desired subjects for the state continued from the previous regime, the curriculum content shifted to meet Japan's imperialist goals. In 1911, the GGK passed the Education Ordinance, setting forth the policies and direction for public education, revised again in 1922, 1938, and 1943. The purpose of education was primarily "to be the making of loyal and good subjects by giving instruction on the basis of the [Japanese] Imperial Rescript Concerning Education."[37] Public schools were divided into three categories—common, vocational, and professional— with the majority of public schools being normal or common schools at the primary and middle school levels.[38] Often interpreted as a terminal course ("In short, a Common School is not necessarily an institution in which preparatory education for a higher school is given"[39]), colonial period education centered on practical skills "indispensable to daily life" as well as on "engendering national characteristics and the spread of the national language," "national" here meaning Japanese.[40] Primary education thus consisted of elementary Japanese literacy training, moral cultivation, physical education, instructions in the basic tenets of hygiene, and technical skills. Moral training at its heart was to instill values and cultivate civic habits appropriate (i.e., desired) for members of the polity, in this case as Japanese colonial subjects. Unlike in the Japanese metropole, universal education was not a goal in the colony, and tuition was charged at a higher rate for Korean students than for Japanese settler children, accounting in part for the much lower rates of school attendance among Koreans.[41]

There is a general consensus in Korean historiography of the contradictory nature of education in colonial Korea. It was at once liberating, offering new opportunities for limited upward social mobility, and restrictive, relegating Korean students to lower-level tracks that prioritized basic literacy, arithmetic, and technical skills, over higher-level academic and professional training.[42] Colonial period education has also been critiqued as part of the larger GGK policy of assimilation of Koreans as loyal Japanese imperial subjects.[43] As Japan mobilized material and human resources to support its imperialist expansion in the Asia-Pacific in the 1940s, the GGK changed the name of elementary schools from common (*pot'ong*) to citizen/imperial subject (*kungmin*) schools in 1941. Elementary schools now were the site of the intentional cultivation of "Japanese imperial subjects" (*hwangguk sinmin*) who would be steadfast in upholding the Japanese *kokutai* ("national polity").[44] Through strict regulations on private schools and control of curriculums and use of textbooks, the GGK ensured that what schools offered met the standards and agenda of the colonial state. Whether Korean students internalized an understanding of themselves as loyal subjects of the Taehan or as subjects of the Japanese colonial state is less relevant to the discussion here than how the GGK's educational policies structured the choices available to students, for these, in turn, informed the personal and professional choices Koreans would make after graduation.

The future *kungmin* imagined by the Taehan and, to an extent, the Japanese colonial states was on the whole gendered male. This does not mean that women were not conceived of as citizens or subjects but rather that the main targets for the disciplining techniques offered in schools were male. While GGK-run common schools at the primary level consisted of both male and female students, schools before 1910 were sex-segregated.[45] If early conceptions of *kungmin* were as future officials and servants for the state's agenda, then the fact that the Taehan state did not establish a school for girls until 1908, over a decade after establishing a public school system, attests to the general marginalization of women in state citizenship drives. The early government textbooks *Sukhye kiryak* (1895) and *People's Elementary Reader* were written in mixed Chinese-Korean script, based on Chinese classical texts, with an emphasis on moral behavior presented in formats with which students of classical Confucian education were familiar.[46] The figures offered as moral exemplars in the *People's Elementary Reader* were all male, such as King Sejong (r. 1418–1450) and Ŭlchi Mundŏk (fl. ca. 612), who defended the Koguryŏ kingdom against the Sui dynasty. Non-Korean figures whose morality, personal conduct, or other achievements were held up for emulation included former American president James Garfield, Christopher Columbus, George Washington, Confucius, and Genghis Khan.[47]

Illustrations of teachers and students in the ethics textbooks published by the Taehan government during the protectorate, *Common School Morals Textbook* (*Pot'ong hakkyo susinsŏ*, 1907, 4 vols.), were all male. Women, if they appeared in the textbooks at all, served primarily to illustrate proper moral behavior (honesty, charity, treatment of animals, care for one's possessions and health), or habits to avoid (superstition, stealing, bothering others). Moreover, illustrations of women were presented primarily in their capacities as mothers, housewives, and nurses, thereby reinforcing to elementary school students that the service desired from women was to care for the welfare of their family members and communities in their domestic capacities as mothers and housewives. Colonial period primary school ethics textbooks published by the GGK (also titled *Common School Morals Textbook*) were not much different, in fact repeating much of the same lessons as the 1907 textbook in a similar fashion—not surprising given that, by

1907, the Japanese RG had administrative control over the Ministry of Education.[48]

The GGK's first publication of textbooks in 1913 presented similar gendered images, with no illustrations of female students or women in professional occupations or positions of authority. Illustrations of female students finally appeared with the 1922 edition.[49] The very first lesson in the first-grade level 1922 textbook was titled "School," with an image of Korean mothers and fathers leading young children of both sexes to the school gate. The last lesson of first grade also depicted a classroom of both male and female students (but separated on opposite sides of the room). These two lessons with students of both sexes were in the first-grade ethics textbooks of all editions, although illustrations varied slightly in each edition. Lessons with illustrations of male students, however, on the whole outnumbered those of female students. Throughout the textbooks across grade levels, nonstudent males were featured in professional roles such as teacher, inventor, and physician. Females, for the most part, remained portrayed in their familial roles as mothers, grandmothers, or sisters, with the exception of one lesson on philanthropy which featured Florence Nightingale, described below.

This suggests the kinds of gendered citizenship expected of women at this time. Although the Kabo reforms and the "Civilization and Enlightenment" discourse of the late nineteenth century envisioned a social leveling that implicitly assumed women were equal to men as citizens or subjects of the state, male students were prioritized in state-directed civic education. Women were to be incorporated into the polity in ways different than men, and their educations were to account for and reflect those differences. These ideas circulated in the nascent print media. For example, Ch'anyanghoe argued in 1898 that women's education was necessary for the country to stand firmly in the new global order in which it was increasingly incorporated, for it would allow all subjects to "cultivate themselves through learning" and "make [Taehan] an exemplary country in the East and lead [it] to equal treatment with other countries."[50] But the views of how education would help varied. An 1899 editorial in the progressive Christian enlightenment-oriented *Tongnip sinmun* newspaper, "Nyŏ hakkyo ron" [Treatise on girls' schools], explicated that the education of women who made up half of the population would serve as a "benefit to the whole country" by providing children with loving teachers and men with beautiful friends, spreading natural civilization to all corners of the society.[51] Women, whose status was understood as a barometer for the level of civilization achieved in Chosŏn and the basis on which it was judged, were to be "enlightened" and elevated by formal education. Their achievements would impact the world around them through their relations with the men in their families: "If Korean women are admired by other countries . . . [and] well received in the world, will not their sons, brothers, husbands, and fathers also bask in the glory?"[52]

In addition, reformers asserted that the value of girls' schools also lay in their abilities to ensure harmony in the newly idealized household, promoting a domesticity suited for both Christian and nation-building purposes.[53] Schools would cultivate women as partners fit for men who received the new education, ostensibly preventing the breakdown of marriages as it was supposed husbands would tire of ignorant wives.[54] Such a result would weaken the moral fabric of a social order based on the notion of Korea as a community of households under the benevolent rule of the monarch. Moreover, the new domestic management required knowledge and skills that the new-style education could offer female students.

But perhaps the most compelling reason offered for providing schools for girls was the need to produce learned mothers who would apply their education in the raising of future citizens: "they will know how to raise and teach their children, and in this way the children will grow up to be useful. . . . Hence, women's duty is no less than that of men: the future citizens of the country are totally in the hands of women."[55] Christian education, too, focused on the reproductive role of women. According to Ji-Eun Lee, it comes as little surprise that editorials regarding women in *Tongnip sinmun* revolved around two main themes: women's domestic roles and their education.[56]

The positioning of women in their communities or the state in roles as housewives and mothers was enabled by new notions of the home and, accordingly, the family, domestic work, and household management. "Home," as it evolved in the early twentieth century, was tempered by Chosŏn conventions, missionaries' understandings of domesticity, and Japanese concepts encapsulated by the neologism *kajŏng* (家庭; J. *katei*). According to Jordan Sand, Meiji reformers used the Chinese characters for "household" and "garden" to define the home as a domestic space that was "an arena for social reform" as well as "an environment, a family group, and a set of practices."[57] The term *kajŏng* was adapted by Koreans but did not take root immediately or initially signify the "intimate space sequestered from society and centered on parents and children" that *katei* idealized in Japan.[58] *Kajŏng* could refer to the conjugal space of home but was often understood in the broader sense of *ka* or household as it did in earlier times, referencing the estate and extended family relations, as well as servants, or even clan and lineage. *Kajŏng* was also used as a modifier with concepts such as "education" (*kajŏng kyoyuk*, "education in the home") or "hygiene" (*kajŏng wisaeng*, "hygiene in the home").

Furthermore, *kajŏng* was not necessarily gendered at first. When used with education, *kajŏng* merely pointed to the importance of the home as the first site of education, one that formed moral children's habits and values and provided future citizens with civic education.[59] The role of teacher or implementer of *kajŏng kyoyuk*, was not limited to mothers. For example, the academic society *Sŏbuk Hakhoe* in 1909 stated that the early education of children was to be a cooperative effort among family members, including both father and mother.[60] The morals textbook *Ch'odŭng susinsŏ* (Elementary morals) published by Pak Chŏngdong that same year for use in private schools, illustrated the lesson "Kajŏng kyoyuk" (sec. 1, chap. 3) with an image of a father presiding over the early education of his three children.[61] Over time, however, *kajŏng*'s meaning solidified to refer to home or family. It also became gendered female, associated specifically with and under the charge of married women, and as such was used in the titles of journals such as *Kajŏng chapchi* (Home Journal, 1906–1908) or *Sin kajŏng* (New Home, 1933–1936), and special sections or columns in colonial-era newspapers such as *Kajŏng puinnan* (Housewives' column) in the *Chosŏn ilbo* that aimed to provide married women with new knowledge resonant with the household-related curriculum.

Social expectations for women in their dual roles as mothers and household managers became expressed in the neologism Wise Mother, Good Wife (*hyŏnmo yangch'ŏ*), which was at the core of a new gender discourse in Korea in the early twentieth century through its institution in girls' schools. The term was adapted from the Japanese ideal of modern womanhood, denoted by Good Wife, Wise Mother (J. *ryōsai kenbo*), which conjured Confucian values associated with classical female virtues.[62] Yet *ryōsai kenbo* was in fact a Meiji creation designed to promote what was perceived as the proper sexual division of labor in the modern era, with men working outside the home and women relegated to housework and child-rearing. The Meiji state promoted women's roles as mothers who raised healthy and loyal children, wives who supported their husbands, and household managers whose economic activities would contribute to Japan's industrialization and military exploits.[63] Accordingly, it instituted *ryōsai kenbo* as the mission and function of female education with the 1895 Provision of Girls' High Schools, which also stipulated the curriculum and number of years of study.[64] Meiji schools for girls valorized practical skills that would be employed in their future households and workplaces while maintaining what were deemed the traditional merits of Japanese women.

The Wise Mother, Good Wife ideal became institutionalized in public schools of the colonial period. That the GGK differentiated education between the sexes is evident in its ethics textbooks. Each edition included in grade-level textbooks a lesson that defined male duties and female duties. The 1913 edition for Grade 4 (Lesson 22), for example, states that a man is to be master in his house, devote himself to his work, and contribute to the family, while a woman is to keep house, support her husband, serve his parents, and raise the children she bears. Moreover, as the influence of a mother on the education of her children is large, whether they become good *kungmin* depends on her. The 1922 edition for Grade 6 (Lesson 6) further explicates that while men and women are both *kungmin*, how they fulfill their roles differs due to their physiological differences. The stronger of the two, men are to defend their houses, society, and country, whereas women are to ensure peace and joy at home while serving their parents-in-law and raising children. Fulfilling their duties strengthens the country.

According to Hyaeweol Choi, the Wise Mother, Good Wife construct in Korea emerged as an inflection of Korean, Japanese imperial, and Protestant Christian visions of domesticity and womanhood, also formalized through girls' schools.[65] Like the earlier Chosŏn female primers discussed in the last section, Wise Mother, Good Wife premised the domestic space as the rightful locus of women's work and responsibilities. As an idealized vision of womanhood, it demarcated status in twentieth-century Korea. *Pudŏk* as prescribed among the elite during the

Chosŏn period had revolved around one's position and relations in the household, directing how a woman was to behave and what roles she was to perform.[66] The Wise Mother, Good Wife model presented in the early twentieth century distinguished the privileged, educated, middle- and upper-class minority, from the working and rural majority who lacked the requisite material means and academic achievements to implement the tenets of or become themselves a Wise Mother, Good Wife.[67] Finally, whereas in Chosŏn idealized womanhood was cultivated by the mastering of instructions and virtues presented in selected Confucian classics and household handbooks, the linking of early twentieth-century girls' schools to diverse goals that supported national strengthening and survival, the Japanese imperial system, and Christian religious piety began to shift female curriculum away, though not entirely, from the moral tenor of Chosŏn primers and toward modern visions of science. This is demonstrated in the cluster of household-related curriculum *kajŏnghak* as it evolved in the early twentieth century.

WISAENG IN MORAL INSTRUCTION

The history of the academic discipline *kajŏnghak*, or home economics, in Korea is often described as starting with the new mission girls' schools of the 1890s, such as Ewha Girls' School, which assigned housekeeping tasks to students in the dormitories and cafeteria and later introduced classes on sewing, embroidery, and cooking.[68] *Kajŏnghak*, however, also took shape through private textbook publications and state promulgations on women's education. Both drew heavily from Japanese models that Jordan Sand describes as an eclectic discipline with roots in Tokugawa moral texts and merchant house codes as well as the home economics curriculum used in Western nations, particularly the United States.[69] This accounts in part for the subject's ambiguous relations with Confucian didactics at the same time it presented itself as a modern subject. Incorporated into the educational system initially on an ad hoc basis and later systematically during the colonial period, various terms besides *kajŏnghak*, including *sallim* (housekeeping) and *kasa* (household matters), were used to indicate a gendered household-related curriculum.

The GGK designated *kasa* as the official name for the female curriculum "home economics."

While *kajŏng* (J. *kasei*) in *kajŏnghak* sounds phonetically similar to *kajŏng* (J. *katei*) that was used to translate home or family in the Korean language, the two were based on different Chinese characters and meanings: "management" and "garden," respectively. As a curriculum, *kajŏnghak/kaseigaku* referenced methods specific to the tasks and principles involved in the management of the home and household, while *kajŏng/katei* was the locus of those operations. Initially, some Korean writers used the two *kajŏng* interchangeably by adding the "learning" Chinese character (*–hak*) to *kajŏng/katei*. Such issues in translation indicate a flux in language at a time when concepts of "home" and "household management" were still being defined.[70] Coupled with the moralist and civic orientation of education in general, the development of *kajŏnghak* reveals interesting shifts in the perception, intention, formulation, and implementation of girls' schools.

Although the Taehan government did not immediately establish a public girls' school in response to Ch'anyanghoe's 1898 petition, it did set aside money in its budget for a girls' school and instituted its Regulation on Girls' Schools in 1899.[71] Budgetary concerns and conservative opposition within the bureaucracy may have sidelined public schooling for girls, but the 1899 Regulation laid the groundwork by establishing the purpose and recommending the curriculum of girls' schools. In the first article, the Regulation stipulated that students learn the knowledge and skills necessary for the development of their bodies and *sallim*, which could mean making a living but in the context of women's education meant housekeeping.[72] This is similar to the stated purpose of education for boys except that the course of study for girls included sewing, in addition to the general curriculum of arithmetic, geography, Korean history, natural sciences, and drawing.[73] Girls were also to learn how to read and exercise their bodies. How this was to be accomplished, however, was left to schools to determine so long as they used textbooks published or approved by the Ministry of Education. Elementary education was to be a three-year course with two years at a higher level, the age level of students restricted to between the ages of nine and fifteen. Boys' schools, in contrast, offered three years at the lower level but also three to four at the middle level with more schooling at higher levels and higher limits on the ages of students.[74] Separate ethics textbooks for girls appeared, further indicating a general understanding that female students were to be taught differently—in theory the same values but applied differently. Published privately, these textbooks mainly modeled moral primers from the Chosŏn period, especially in the use of the exemplary biographies.

The Taehan state's Ministry of Education did not publish or compile a textbook for every subject but relied on private publications to supplement state-produced textbooks. For kajŏnghak, the state approved for use in schools textbooks by well-known translator Hyŏn Kongnyŏm, Hanmun kajŏnghak (Kajŏnghak, Classical Chinese, 1907) and Sinp'yŏn kajŏnghak (Kajŏnghak, New edition, 1907) in classical Chinese and mixed script, respectively.[75] Hyŏn's textbooks were based on what were purportedly Chinese translations of the lectures and writings of Shimoda Utako, an administrator of the Peeresses' School for Girls in Japan, founder of Jissen Jogakkō (The Women's Practical Arts School) and Joshi Kōgei Gakkō (The Women's Industrial Arts School), and supporter of Chinese students studying in Japan.[76] A champion of ryōsai kenbo as the basis for female education, Shimoda firmly believed that women should learn formal job skills to enable their financial contributions to themselves, their families, and their country, while maintaining their major responsibility and explicit role of running the household, the foundation for a well-ordered state.[77] Female students should receive instruction in both general education and vocational training and then apply their scientific skills later as household managers or in the professional realm of business, industrial arts, teaching, or nursing. Shimoda's lectures were published in Japan as Kaseigaku (Household management, 1899), which was revised and reprinted as Shinsen kaseigaku (New household management, 1902). Another approved Korean kajŏnghak textbook of this period, Sinch'an kajŏnghak (Kajŏnghak, New composition, 1907) by Pak Chŏngdong, was a near translation of part of Shimoda's textbooks. In any case, it is evident that Korean writers had access to both Japanese and Chinese texts on kajŏnghak.

Although translations, these textbooks and the extrapolations they inspired suggest the ways Korean reformers conceived and began to implement a female curriculum that included kajŏnghak. As Lydia Liu reminds us, translations are acts of "translingual practices," complex processes that involve agency and negotiations.[78] It was common practice that privately published textbooks or topical treatises in journals of academic societies at this time were based on translations of foreign texts.[79] Translators would sometimes add their own opinions in the text, rearrange chapters, remove or add sections so, in this sense, their texts were not necessarily direct translations of the original source.[80] Examining how and what was translated and the ensuing circulation of the results reveals Koreans' concerns with regard to the education of women.

Kajŏnghak in these early texts reaffirmed the "womanly virtues" of *pudŏk* in Chosŏn household manuals and female texts. In particular, they prioritized women's functions in managing the domestic sphere and the human relations within it. For the most part, this is attributable to the original Japanese and Chinese texts themselves. Hyŏn Kongnyŏm's decision to base his translation on the Chinese text as opposed to the original Japanese may have stemmed from his personal language capability or the general preference of Korean translators of this period for Chinese works, especially in the case of ethics textbooks. But there also remains the possibility that Hyŏn chose the Chinese translation over Shimoda's original text because of its differences, particularly changes in the Chinese translation that emphasized Confucian didactics. For example, Hyŏn's translation opens with a major section on a housewife's duties with regard to other household members, particularly in the education and care or nursing of children and elders in rhetoric similar to Chosŏn period female primers. This was followed by the section "Household Etiquette," referring to the customs or traditions of a household or lineage, which does not even exist in Shimoda's text. Only after these moralistic discussions does practical information related to the new knowledge of *wisaeng* and economics appear.[81] In other words, the sections that specify the application of principles of hygiene, science, budgeting, and efficiency to housekeeping tasks of cooking, cleaning, clothing, and shelter, which made up the bulk of the first volume of Shimoda's two-volume textbook, were placed at the end of Hyŏn's translation.[82]

That educators may have been partial to the moral training aspects of female education is corroborated by Pak Chŏngdong's translation, *Sinch'an kajŏnghak*. Pak translated only the second volume of Shimoda's text (the content that was reformulated in the beginning sections of Hyŏn's translations), and he included elements from Hyŏn's "Household Etiquette" section, such as the proper etiquette or protocol to follow when visiting others and receiving guests (kyoje). Other sections in Pak's translation include the moral education and early infant care of children; serving and treating elders or in-laws; nursing sick family members; handling threats to the house such as natural disasters, thieves, and fires; and the selection and management of servants. Although organized differently, both Pak's and Hyŏn's textbooks share attention to the duties and relations a woman was to have toward members of her husband's household, including her children. The explication of women's responsibilities as mothers and daughters-in-law in preserving the customs, etiquette, property, and descendants of her husband's lineage reflected a continuing propensity toward moral education in female education.

The prominence of moral instruction in female education is reflected in other textbooks for female students published privately at this time. Textbooks such as *Ch'odŭng yŏhak tokpon* (Elementary girls' reader, 1908), *Yŏja sohak susinsŏ* (Girls' elementary moral primer, 1909), and *Yŏja tokpon* (Female primer, 1908) delineated the social roles women should perform with exemplary biographies.[83] The textbooks, however, continued to draw from Chosŏn female texts and promoted an ideal womanhood within the marked boundaries of Confucian "womanly virtues." For example, *Yŏja sohak susinsŏ* instructed women in their roles specifically as new daughters-in-law (chap. 14), wives (chaps. 15–19), mothers (chaps. 20–22), and mothers-in-law (chap. 23).[84] It also included chapters titled, "Gentle Manners" (yamjŏn), "Formal Proprieties" (yejŏl), and "Three Bonds and Five Relationships" (samgang kwa oryun). Schools then were envisioned as the site where a girl would learn how to become a good "mother, mother-in-law, daughter-in-law, sister-in-law, and daughter."[85]

Another point of continuity between Chosŏn period texts and early *kajŏnghak* and ethics textbooks was the importance placed on the home or household, which was organically linked to the state, serving as its foundation. The administration of the country depended on the proper management of individual households. But unlike in the Chosŏn period when men had responsibilities in the management and maintenance of harmony in the household, in twentieth-century textbooks men were removed from household management. Household management became gendered female, now identified as the heavenly ordained duty, responsibility, and civic role of married women.[86] The state of a country's moral character, its financial status, its health, and peace, continued to depend on the moral education learned at home, harmonious relations among household members, maintenance of family appearances and customs, and budgeting of the household's consumption.

A shift, however, began. Added to the duties and tasks of women as part of their proper management of households was *wisaeng*, which referenced the new sanitary and public health practices mobilized for nation-building purposes that Ruth Rogaski calls "hygienic modernity." According to Todd Henry, *wisaeng* as concept and practice also became incorporated into the broad category of *kongdŏk* or "civic morality" that Japanese colonial administrators demanded of Korean colonial subjects in the imperial project of assimilation.[87] Missionaries, too, promoted healthy habits, including temperance and nonsmoking, as part of a Christian lifestyle. Early twentieth-century textbooks and writings for women reformulated the home such that while its stability remained important for the social world beyond, it was also correlated to the housewife's ability to care for the health of members of her household, a goal to which *wisaeng* was indispensable. *Wisaeng* principles shaped the ways a woman would perform her household tasks—the raising of a child, nursing the sick, feeding the family, airing the rooms, clothing bodies, etc. The two principles of frugality (*kyŏngje*) and efficiency (*hyoyul*) that came to the fore in Japanese literature on women's domestic work and colonial Korean discussions later in the 1930s were comparatively limited in scope in contrast to the focus on *wisaeng* at this historical moment.

The prominence of hygiene in early twentieth-century ruminations on *kajŏnghak* and other writings on and for women put into sharp relief the convergence among Korean modernist desires for a healthy populace and a reformed domestic space run accordingly by educated women with the ability to manage that altered space. As indicated earlier, *wisaeng* was central to the arsenal reformers hoped to use to secure Korea's sovereignty. Its proper performance was a mark of civilization and way to gain acceptance into the ranks of advanced nations. Foreign observers were quick to note failures to display those qualities, much to the chagrin of Koreans.

Wisaeng was so integral to the nation's self-strengthening purposes that it was woven into the burgeoning education system. For the general student population, *wisaeng* and health-related subjects were taught primarily in three types of textbooks—morals/ethics (*susin/yulli*), physiology/hygiene (*saengnihak/wisaeng*), and the natural sciences (*igwa*)—and in physical education.[88] While moral primers may not seem a likely place for health instruction, by forging an organic link between the health of the individual and the duty required of citizens of a new nation they promoted health in the development of patriotism and moral character. For example, the first chapter in the 1907 textbook *Ch'odŭung yullihak kyogwasŏ* (Elementary ethics) is "Protecting Health."[89] To live in a country means to become a person of that country, and in order to socialize harmoniously with others in that country, people must first refine themselves in the accomplishment of three tasks: (1) protect their health, (2) cultivate their ethics, and (3) broaden their intellect.[90] "Protecting health" here was fused with cleanliness (*ch'ŏnggyŏl*), and drew on the three elements of food, clothing, and shelter. Not only should what one eats, what one wears, and where one lives be clean, but they should also, respectively, be nourishing, protective (guarding against climatic elements), and safe. Bad habits, such as excessive alcohol consumption and irregular eating, bring disease and weakness, which has direct ramifications for the state. A weak country is weak because its youth are ignorant in the ways of physical education (*ch'eyuk*), the lesson exhorts. Loving one's country, then, requires individuals to combat their physical weakness. This is the health citizenship that the initiated student was to learn and practice.

Morals and ethics textbooks continued throughout the colonial period to teach lessons on the merits of *wisaeng*, instilling healthy habits of exercise and cleanliness and encouraging proper medical care.[91] While in their science courses, students were to learn about human anatomy and physiological functions of the body as a basis for health instruction, on the whole *wisaeng* directives in related textbooks remained theoretical or vague—keep clean, avoid alcohol, exercise regularly, maintain a calm composure, avoid indigestion with frequent but small meals, etc.[92] Government ethics textbooks in the protectorate and colonial period also reinforced certain health habits. For example, in

Lesson 11, "Body," of the first-grade level of the RG period ethics text-book, students learned that one had to take care of one's body because worrying one's parents by getting sick would be the most unfilial act. Falling ill, the lesson continued, often resulted from not keeping the body clean, eating unripened or rotten fruit, or not exercising suffi-ciently. Lessons on keeping one's clothes, possessions, and public facili-ties clean and being careful what one ate continued in GGK-published ethics textbooks.[93] Just as RG and GGK ethics textbooks were oriented generally toward the male student, lessons related to *wisaeng* also were presented in slightly gendered ways. For example, in most of these les-sons, those who practiced *wisaeng* as it affected others (visiting a sick friend, caring for a sick child, washing the hair or clipping the nails of another, warning others to stay away from harmful food or refrain from spoiling the public drinking well, laundering clothes so they stay clean, scrubbing the floors) were female.[94] Boys too were illustrated engaged in health-promoting behavior but primarily when it affected their indi-vidual bodies (such as washing one's self or being vaccinated).[95] Caring for others was acceptable for a male as an act of filial piety (such as giv-ing medicine to an ailing mother under the supervision of an older sis-ter) or in the role of a professional physician.

Similar ideas pervaded discussions and texts for female education. The happiness of a woman's household and hence the happiness of her country depended on her ability to economize in household finances, preserve family customs, and properly supervise household members.[96] A woman should protect the heavenly predetermined life span of mem-bers of her household through hygienic principles. This required sin-cere deliberation on how she should make clothes and clothe herself and others (appropriate to seasons and weather), prepare and store food (clean and nourishing), and maintain a salubrious home environment (ensure sufficient ventilation, reduce humidity levels, etc.). She was also to see that her children received the proper vaccinations. As the primary overseer of the health of her family, she was to be equipped with new knowledge in medicine and hygiene, even perhaps to follow the path of Florence Nightingale and become a nurse.[97] Information relating to these matters became a frequent feature in print media, particularly those targeting a female readership such as the journals *Kajŏng chapchi*

(Home Journal) and *Chasŏn puinhoe chapchi* (Journal of Women's Society for Charity).

The change in the understanding of women's roles with respect to the raising of children is especially evident when the prescriptions for women in the early twentieth century are contrasted with the concerns expressed in Chosŏn period household manuals. As discussed earlier, child-rearing per se took up marginal space in Chosŏn female texts and tended to be curt, focusing on techniques to conceive and ensure the successful gestation and delivery of male children based on Sino-classical medical cosmologies of correspondence and morality. Little attention was paid to instructions on how to provide for the physical and mental health of children, except in terms of simple admonitions to instill moral conduct in children or general first-aid procedures. In contrast, the new *kajŏnghak* texts, while still highly moral in tone, stressed a woman's role as mother and offered concrete instructions on Western child-rearing techniques based on modernist principles of hygiene to practice in everyday life. The *kajŏnghak* texts, for example, introduced new breastfeeding principles such as feeding on schedule and not on demand, not falling asleep when breastfeeding at night for fear of crushing the baby to death, eating appropriately to avoid indigestion, and preparing milk formula to supplement insufficient breast milk.[98] Other new instructions included using antisepsis to cleanse wounds, inducing vomiting after the ingestion of spoiled food, and bathing the sick. Women were to consult a hospital, a novelty at this time, if warranted.[99]

The overall narrative in female education was that the person mainly entrusted with *wisaeng* directives in day-to-day tasks were women as mothers and housewives, for the home was the primary site (as the place where one would eat, sleep, bathe, etc.) of *wisaeng* performance.[100] Caring for, fostering habits in, and making health decisions for children fell primarily to mothers. Female students were required not only to learn the general principles of *wisaeng* but had to learn more of it than male students, and also its specific applications.[101] As we will see, *wisaeng* instructions were inserted throughout the curriculum during the colonial period, from the posture girls were to take in their physical education class to ethics and housekeeping instructions (cooking, nursing, clothing/textiles) in *kasa* courses.[102]

KAJŎNGHAK: FROM MORAL
TO PRACTICAL ARTS

Hygiene instruction for female students surged during the colonial period, reflecting the development of home economics at higher levels of education. After Japan formalized Korea as a colony, the term *kajŏnghak* was no longer commonly used, as *kasagwa* ("the subject of *kasa*") became the official term to designate this curriculum, as in Japan. *Kasa*, as it became standardized in Korea, did not include sewing and handicrafts, which were separated as autonomous subjects, but instead assembled increasingly technical instructions for housekeeping that contributed to the construction of a new womanhood centered around women's roles as mothers and housewives. Offered at secondary school institutions beyond the primary common schools, *kasa* courses drew from Japanese and American models.

Efforts in the United States to make home economics at the college and graduate level an academic discipline that employed recent developments in social and natural sciences to train women for professional work in the "municipal home" beyond the four walls of their individual homes, failed to persuade elite East Coast women's colleges to accept home economics in their liberal arts curriculum.[103] Instead, home economics at the college level was relegated to vocational training, paralleling for women the practical courses for men in animal husbandry and agriculture developed in the land-grant colleges of the United States. Science remained an integral part of the home economics curriculum but primarily insofar as it was applicable to productive or occupational work. Korea's household-related curriculum intersected with science in similar ways as its development drew significantly from American models and experiences filtered through Japan and foreign missionaries.[104] Pioneering home economics educators in Japan such as Shimoda Utako; Miyakawa Sumi, professor of *kaji* at the Department of Art and Craft at Home at Tokyo Women's Higher Normal School; and Inoue Hide, dean of Home Economics at the Japan Women's Institute (*Nihon joshi daigaku*), studied American and British programs on official trips. While they may have differed in their pedagogical visions in regard to home economics (technical training vs. interdisciplinary sciences), they generally agreed on the incorporation of sciences in relation to their practical use.[105]

If science is to be understood as the study of the natural world, then science education was not unfamiliar to Koreans, having existed as part of a broader Confucian curriculum.[106] But in the face of global pressures and transformation, the sciences increasingly took on a different meaning of knowledge gained through observation and experimentation. Students were to come to know "truth" (sasil) through observation (mokkyŏk). The purpose of experiments was to help students understand what they were observing. The Board of Education as early as 1895 defined the sciences as that which related to the material phenomena of the natural world of plants and animals.[107] Chemistry and physics as they related to plant and animal life, and physiology and hygiene as they related to human bodies, thus were included in the category of the sciences. In fact, it was the biological sciences (with earth science as a close second) that were most represented among scientific treatises published by academic societies in Korea between 1905 and 1910.[108] Notably, wisaeng and physiology accounted for the majority of these biology-related treatises.

Associations of science with contemplation of the operations and metaphysics of the cosmos, however, were not yet completely severed. In 1906, an article in the publication of the academic society Sŏbuk Hakhoe clarified science (kwahak) as the learning of systematic theories or principles, including those of nature, phenomenology, and human activity and organization. Accordingly, it included physics, chemistry, physiology, geology, zoology, and botany along with psychology, philosophy, law, and economics.[109] Over time, this became expressed as "scientism," a valorization of that which was declared "science" or "scientific" and would yield knowledge about the world and man that was true. It was moral in the sense that science naturalized as objective truth could then be applied to benefit society and produce a better future. This was the basis for the Taehan state's "Industrial Promotion Policy" to promote engineering projects and scientific education. Faith in science encouraged incorporation of technical and vocational training in public education. In the 1906 revision to the ordinance on normal schools, the Ministry of Education expanded the concept of science education to include industrial (later called vocational) training in the manual arts such as handicrafts and sewing, agriculture, fisheries, and housekeeping.[110] The Ministry of Education's inclusion of a household curriculum cemented its relationship with the sciences. For this reason, I include female vocational training under the larger umbrella of the Domestic Sciences. It provided technical training, now understood within the larger rubric of "science," at the same time it drew from diverse categories of scientific knowledge such as *wisaeng* and its related studies in medicine, physiology, biology, chemistry, and psychology.

The GGK juxtaposed vocational with morals training in accord with the direction home economics had taken in Japan but within the circumscribed goals for education conceived by Japanese colonial authorities in Korea. The primary common school level included science and basic industrial or crafts training, which, although provided to both boys and girls, were gendered in that "these should be taught correspondingly to the natural propensities of boys and girls."[111] Boys were taught manual skills that could be applied to the rural or industrial sector, such as techniques in drawing/drafting, elementary agriculture, and elementary commerce. Girls learned sewing and other handicrafts that might or might not overlap with boys' industrial training. Initially, these courses in manual work, handicrafts, and elementary agriculture or commerce were not required but depended on "local conditions."[112]

The more practical orientation to learning extended to the natural sciences. Korean students found they could not pursue advanced science education except in medicine in Korea, and would have to study abroad to fulfill other ambitions in the sciences.[113] As discussed earlier, elementary schools were not to prepare students for higher learning but to "help the cultivation of moral character and the pursuit of daily life" to which the sciences might contribute.[114] Yet, according to *Manual of Education in Chosen* (1920), "science may be dispensed with for the time being."[115] If taught, it would be done so in a way so that students "understand ordinary things and phenomena of nature, their mutual relations and the outline of their relations with human life" so that they may "adapt their knowledge to practical purposes in life . . . which may help them afterwards in pursuing industry and is indispensable in daily life."[116] For this reason equal course time at the elementary level (two hours a week in the fourth year) was allotted for the learning of sciences related to the functioning of the body such as hygiene and physiology, as it was for all other natural sciences relating to plants, animals, minerals, and other natural phenomena.[117] Female students were to study, in addition, "matters concerning house-keeping," categorized under "nature study."[118] In accordance with the moral-practical axis inherent in primary education to "foster in the minds of the pupils the love and habit of steady work and industry,"[119] girls were to learn how to sew with "thrift and utilization" using inexpensive cloth.[120] They also were to cultivate "order and cleanliness."[121] These directives on hygiene and, in later years, efficiency and economy in household management also served to foster the feminine virtues resonant with the Wise Mother, Good Wife ideal.

It was at the higher common (middle school) level that science education and industrial training became required and more pronouncedly gendered. Boys had to study "agriculture or commerce and manual work"; their science courses included natural history, physics, and chemistry, again due to the perceived applicability of these subjects to "industry, law and economy."[122] Girls studied "botany, zoology, human physiology and hygiene, physics and chemistry," subjects which were to "be taught with connections to household matters."[123] Girls could also opt to take a more intensive arts course that specialized in sewing and handicrafts and included use of machines, dyeing, weaving, laundering, tailoring, mending, braid making, pouch making, and artificial flower making; however this was not popular and eventually was phased out.

The GGK did not publish its own set of *kasa* textbooks so girls' high schools in Korea used Japanese *kasa* textbooks that roughly followed the outline of the curriculum presented by Shimoda Utako's early *kaseigaku* textbook, with two volumes divided into units consisting of clothing and textiles, food and nutrition, and housing and habitat in the first volume; and basic nursing, child-rearing, and household budgeting and management in the second.[124] High schools for girls were to produce morally principled and technically skilled housekeepers ("modest and faithful women of industrial and thrifty disposition").[125] Accordingly, courses in *kasa* and sewing-handicrafts served as vocational courses for girls in the way that instruction in agriculture, commerce, or manual work served male students. This did not necessarily mean that female graduates received vocational training through which they could seek paid employment postgraduation, although some did.[126] Primarily it justified the large proportion of hours of classroom instruction devoted to the

Domestic Sciences, and hence, by default, science defined very broadly. In fact, girls were allotted more class time for sciences and skills training than boys. Teachers were instructed by the educational ordinances that in girls' schools "comparatively . . . more hours have been allotted to the teaching of such subjects as natural sciences, housekeeping, sewing and handicraft, and the method of using sewing machines."[127] Hours devoted to Domestic Sciences courses occupied between 33 percent and nearly 50 percent of the curriculum in girls' higher school education depending on whether the specialized arts course was taken, *kasa* being thus the most important subject for girls, following Japanese language.[128] The sciences in general became so much more important to the girls' curriculum that in later revisions to the educational ordinance of 1911, time allotted for natural sciences was increased by an hour per week.[129]

One significant contrast in science education between boys and girls was the way physiology was taught. Physiology textbooks on the whole explained in technical terms the functioning of different systems in the human body such as the respiratory, circulatory, and digestive systems, accompanied with illustrations. What was notably absent, however, was the reproductive system—this was the case in Japanese as well as colonial Taiwanese textbooks.[130] The physiology of the reproductive system was, as expected, taught in medical courses, or published privately in the general print media. It was not taught regularly in high school physiology classes. However, girls' high schools taught the physiology of pregnancy through *kasa* textbooks in the unit on child-rearing.[131]

While the focus of the child-rearing unit was the development and care of young infants (including breastfeeding and common pediatric ailments), students learned what changes to expect in their bodies, precautions they should take to protect the health of themselves and their unborn child, preparations for home delivery, as well as how to care for their reproductive bodies, particularly the menstrual cycle and the factors affecting it.[132] This perhaps reflected a tradition of household primers and pre-1910 *kajŏnghak* textbooks that began with instructions in prenatal *t'aegyo* education. It was also likely permissible based on the logic that science education for girls was to operate in relation to household matters. If the child-rearing unit in *kasa* depended on the birth of and care for healthy infants, which fed into the biopolitics of the Japanese colonial state, female students must know and understand their reproductive bodies in order to be healthy reproducers and nurturers of their future children. The absence of discussion of the male reproductive system in boys' high school textbooks further solidified the removal of men from reproductive functions and responsibilities. This is in contrast to Chosŏn period medical and household texts that included instructions for men in conception and the prenatal care of fetuses. While the male reproductive system was discussed in colonial period newspapers and journals, those articles often targeted female readers who needed to understand the physiology and psychology of their pubescent sons. The exclusion of the reproductive system from high school physiology courses also suggests the relative reluctance of the GGK and Japanese imperial government to include sex education or sexology for male secondary school students.

Concern with *wisaeng* further intensified in the colonial period. Hygienic principles were included in nearly every unit of *kasa* courses. Instructions on dyeing clothes black related to the assertion that black clothing was more hygienic and appropriate for "lifestyle improvement" (*saenghwal kaesŏn*).[133] A woman was to choose architectural elements in her family's residence and implement cleaning routines in consideration of hygienic principles. Menus were to be planned to maximize nutritional value and prepared in a hygienic manner. Naturally, the raising of children and nursing the sick also were guided by *wisaeng*. These two were significant components of *kasa* and fostered modern womanhood's orientation toward caring for members of the household. Based on Chŏn Migyŏng's survey of several *kasa* textbooks used in the 1930s, units on nursing and child-rearing took up at least 70 percent of the second volume.[134]

The inclination of the state and educators to view *wisaeng* instructions as perhaps more important for women than men was also shared by foreign missionaries. Medical services were a central component of the Protestant mission enterprise in Korea, not only for the access to potential converts they provided but also as an expression of Christian charity and the Christian lifestyle. From their early years of activity in Korea, missionaries actively incorporated health education and services in their programs, instructing from the pulpit and publishing tracts on hygiene. A 1909 report of the Presbyterian Caroline A. Ladd Hospital in Pyongyang declared that Dr. J. H. Wells' publication *Introduction to*

Hygiene was a most popular seller.[135] Missionaries incorporated hygiene education in their Bible Training Institutes and Bible Women's training, but female students had additional science courses related to hygiene compared to male students. The Presbyterian Theological Seminary did not teach physiology at all to its male students.[136]

The emphasis on hygiene education for women in particular spilled over into the public spaces of print media. When examining women's columns in newspapers and women's journals of 1920s and 1930s Korea, two terms or phrases emerge repeatedly in the various articles on house-hold tasks: *ŭi-sik-chu* ("clothing, food, residence") and *wisaeng*, both of which reflect the general contours of the *kasa* curriculum. While not specifically targeting a female audience, editorials related to family life in the daily newspaper *Maeil sinbo* were most numerous on hygiene-related topics, particularly in the 1910s and early 1920s, with the focus turning to child-rearing in the 1920s and 1930s.[137] This corresponds with the GGK's interest to promote its new charity hospitals and public health initiatives in the 1910s and its "lifestyle improvement" and infant welfare campaigns of the 1930s—not surprising, since the *Maeil sinbo* served basically as the mouthpiece of the GGK. This emphasis in print media on hygiene and child-rearing was also reflected in the "House-wives' Column" (*Kajŏng puinnan*) of the daily newspaper *Chosŏn ilbo*. The *Tonga ilbo* hired physicians to write on medical-*wisaeng* issues in relation to the home and women.[138] Even informal education for women in night schools, factories, and mothers' clubs in rural areas or those affiliated with kindergartens or churches included hygiene instruction as a central part of their curriculum.

Very few women had access to primary much less high school educa-tion. Even fewer had the resources, fortitude, or family support to go further. Initial attendance at girls' schools was low, but over time more and more families sent their daughters to receive elementary and even higher education. Many contemporaries were critical of higher female education, particularly in that they perceived it as being impractical and inaccessible to the majority of Korean households. By 1919, only 5,008 female students attended normal school, with a dismal gradua-tion rate of 18.7 percent.[139] Two decades later (1937), the number had risen to 64,809, less than one-third the number of male students, but with a higher graduation rate of about 73.7 percent.[140] Education for women had inherent contradictions. On the one hand, education provided women with skills that presented opportunities for them to participate publicly in society in ways they were unable to before, such as traveling abroad, producing work in literary publications, or financially supporting themselves as professionals. On the other hand, female education idealized women's role in the now designated private spaces of the family and home. This in turn placed limits on the educational, occupational, and lifestyle opportunities available to women. Female education, it appeared, served foremost to produce mothers and housekeepers who met nationalist, imperial, and Christian directives outfitted with what was perceived as advanced scientific principles and skills.

The formal education of women nevertheless became a permanent fixture of the Korean landscape. The Domestic Sciences, which included *kasa*, sewing-handicrafts, cooking, and other related sciences was solidified as part of a legitimate and standardized education for female students, particularly at the high school and college levels. Before 1945, with limited opportunities for professional learning available for women in the sciences, a degree in *kasa* was an acceptable alternative for ambitious women and could lead to professional opportunities in teaching or social welfare. *Kasa* was in fact the most popular major chosen by female students studying abroad in Japan.[141] Many returning after their studies became *kasa* teachers at the primary and high school levels.

Kasa also grew quickly as a department at Ewha College after its establishment in 1929.[142] Its graduates went on to work as educators and administrators in Christian or social service organizations. Oregon Agricultural College offered scholarships for Ewha graduates to receive postgraduate training in home economics in the United States. Recipients, such as Kim Hamna, Kim Punok, and Ch'oe Yisun, frequently returned to Korea to join the faculty of their alma mater.[143] However, *kasa* in Korea lacked the impetus for women's professionalization that was present in the American home economics movement. Two of the department chairs at Ewha, Kim Hamna and Mable Kim, left their positions upon marriage. On the whole, the purpose of higher education in the Domestic Sciences was foremost to train future mothers and housewives and provide temporary professional opportunities for single women.

Moreover, the sciences, particularly those in the household-related curriculum, remained more applied than professional or research-oriented in this period. A degree in *kasa* was a worthy alternative to a science-based curriculum that was basically unavailable to women. Before 1945, although the program at Ewha required students to take high-level science courses, and hired medical and science PhDs to teach courses on sanitation, physiology, and bacteriology, a degree in *kasa* did not prepare young women for careers in the sciences or health care. Students conducted experiments in the laboratory but these were to calculate the caloric and nutritional value of foods to confirm the viability of menu plans. The "Practice Home" gave seniors the opportunity to try their learned skills in modern housekeeping and child care before graduating. Chemistry in relation to dye making allowed students to create textiles and clothing that would not physically harm the body. The true purpose of modern principles of science and efficiency was to "separate the new domestic knowledge from the old" and thereby shift women's education from one that emphasized a woman's responsibilities to the preservation of the property and practices of her husband's lineage toward the acquisition of technical skills that would enable successful household management to protect her family's health in the absence of comprehensive public health services and promote frugality and efficiency.

More importantly, *kasa* and by extension the Domestic Sciences were promoted as the means to provide stable peaceful homes as an antidote to social problems. Men who stayed out drinking and consorting with female entertainers, high rates of infant mortality, and concubinage were perceived as some of the problems that arose when housewives failed to create a home environment that taught morality and produced virtuous people. The Domestic Sciences, with its twin technical and moral agendas, had the intent to empower women with the skills to construct a home that would serve as a haven from the external threats of stress and disease; develop family members, especially children, so that they might contribute productively to society; and ensure societal stability with secure families. In short, as Kim Hamna, chair of Ewha's *kasa* department asserted, the Domestic Sciences in general and home economics in particular allowed female education "to meet exigencies of Korean home life in a scientific way."[144]

Science education then was requisite for women, perhaps best displayed by the ways the Domestic Sciences intersected with the modernist desires to promote health in Korea. Instructions in health and the sciences, particularly physiology and hygiene, became increasingly central to the curriculum in girls' schools and prominent in print media that targeted female readers, to both of which scholars attribute the scientification of the domestic realm and the medicalization of child-rearing. What teaching hygiene to women hinged on foremost was their future or present roles as mothers. Women were to "sanitize" their homes by applying *wisaeng* principles in housekeeping tasks and the preparation of food and clothing. They were also to instill healthy habits such as bathing, exercise, sleeping sufficiently, and receiving proper medical attention when indicated. By so doing, they could "sanitize" their family members, especially their children, and potentially ward off or at least successfully manage serious disease. Ultimately, the Domestic Sciences re-imagined and reinforced expectations for women. If citizenship is understood as a cultural ideal, "infused with moral meaning, encompassed by normative principles, values, and expectations," and not simply in terms of rights and entitlements, then a major way women exercised their citizenship was premised on their increased health literacy and activities as mothers and guardians of the health of their families.[145] This care-providing role also laid the foundations for the professionalization of women's medical work.

CHAPTER 2

From the *Ŭinyŏ* to the *Yŏ'ŭi*

The Female Physician

In 1886, Horace Allen, Presbyterian missionary and attendant physician of the royal hospital Chejungwŏn, reported that he had difficulty treating Korean women of high rank because of the strict rules of decorum mandating that their travel to the hospital as well as their physical examination be "perfectly private."[1] To rectify this, his request for female medical assistants was granted by the court, which provided young girls, whom Allen described as belonging to the "'Dancing Girl' order," whose low status allowed them freer mobility and contact with both sexes. Allen designated these girls "medical students" and expected them to "lead pure lives and become nurses." But, as he later recalled in his journal, they continued to perform entertainment functions for dignitaries, serving wine and playing music.[2] In the end, he deemed it necessary to remove them from their positions.

When Allen subsequently reported that "a hospital for women is a necessity," missionary societies responded by commissioning female medical missionaries to Korea and funding medical work for Korean women. Trained nurse Annie J. Ellers of the Presbyterian Board arrived later that year to assist in medical work with women at Chejungwŏn and at the palace and was succeeded two years later by Dr. Lillias S. Horton.[3] In 1887, the Woman's Foreign Missionary Society (WFMS) of the Methodist Episcopal Church (MEC) sent Dr. Meta Howard, who taught at the new mission Ewha Girls' School and was instrumental in the 1888 founding of the hospital Pogunyŏgwan that aimed primarily to serve female patients with female physicians.[4] This facility, which in 1912 was incorporated into the Lillian Harris Memorial Hospital—known to

Koreans as East Gate Women's Hospital—cultivated Korea's first female nurses and physicians.[5]

The difficulties that missionaries initially faced in their schools in recruiting, training, and retaining Korean female personnel were replicated and intensified in their medical institutions. While the Chosŏn state had implemented a centralized system that selected, educated, and employed *ŭinyŏ* (醫女), female medical practitioners, in various state institutions, the *ŭinyŏ*'s association with the lowest *ch'ŏnmin* status group rendered medicine an unattractive occupation for women, especially if it combined the entertaining functions for the state that Horace Allen observed. Thus, Korean women with whom medical missionaries worked in the early period were predominantly widows, disabled, or with other marginal statuses.[6] While some Korean Christian families permitted medical training for their daughters, those women often left due to marriage or other domestic demands. The gendered customs in Korea that discouraged female higher education and work outside the home after marriage long frustrated missionary efforts to train female medical workers, whether as assistants, nurses, or physicians.[7] In 1910, there were only twenty registered Korean female midwives, seventeen nurses, and one physician.[8]

By the 1920s, however, trained and licensed female physicians, nurses, and midwives had gained employment in hospitals and clinics, opened private practices, participated in public health campaigns, published articles on health-related matters, and organized themselves professionally. A 1927 article in the journal *Pyŏlgŏngon* reported that the medical profession headed the list of the most appropriate and desirable occupations for women.[9] Nurses averaged a salary comparable to telephone operators, while midwives and physicians could earn double that.[10] Although there were no official statistics on the number of female physicians, GGK-published statistics reported 135 licensed Korean nurses and 115 midwives for 1927. By 1942, the numbers had increased even more dramatically, to 1,017 nurses and 827 midwives.

This chapter addresses how the health profession became a career choice—albeit a challenging one—for Korean women, by providing an overview of the professionalization of female physicians as it evolved within the public health and medical systems administered by the Taehan state, foreign Protestant missionaries, and, later, the Japanese colonial government. Korean women's participation in medicine in the early twentieth century is best understood when situated in the context of Korean modernist desires, the medical administration of the colonial state, gendered practices, and the professionalization of medical personnel. The complex synergy between constructed notions of womanhood and medicine harbored by foreign missionaries, Japanese colonial authorities, and Korean society shaped the professional experiences of the new female physician or *yŏ'ŭi* (女醫) as she was now called. The medical field granted women expanded educational and occupational opportunities. Yet at the same time, it reinforced gendered labor and spatial divisions, restricting those very opportunities and marginalizing women in medicine at large.

DEFINING THE PHYSICIAN

The emergence of new medical occupations such as physician and nurse at the turn of the twentieth century marked a breaking away from older status designations and the laying of the groundwork for the rise of a new professional elite. As explained in the last chapter, Chosŏn society was status-based and hierarchical, with the highest recognition and privilege awarded to the hereditary *yangban* status group.[11] An official position in the bureaucracy, for which one qualified by one's status and performance in the civil service examination system, was the preferred career for ambitious *yangban* men. Lower-ranked but technically skilled functions in the bureaucracy such as translation, engineering, accounting, law, and the arts were filled by the *chungin* secondary status group, appointment granted through the state *chapkwa* technical exams. In this context, medicine was a craft. The state-employed male medical practitioners worked in state medical organs such as the palace clinic Naeŭiwŏn, reserved for treatment of the royal family and capital-based high-level bureaucrats, and the relief institution Hyeminsŏ.[12] These *chungin* medical practitioners were distinguished from the *yu'ŭi* (Ch. *ruyi*) "scholar-physicians," or members of the male *yangban* elite, whose professed self-cultivation in scholarship and moral behavior valorized their medical knowledge and skills.[13]

The Chosŏn state's system for recruiting, training, and employing *ŭinyŏ* female medical workers was established in the early period of the dynasty primarily to accommodate rules of proper female behavior that restricted women's contact with men. They performed medical functions (diagnosing, distributing medications, physical treatments such as acupuncture or dental work, and some midwifery) throughout the country in various medical, relief, and pharmaceutical institutions.[14] While the medical work they performed was not much different from that of male physicians, the *ŭinyŏ* received a less demanding education, limited to basic medical knowledge and therapeutic techniques. They also lacked comparable authority, having to consult with male superiors who often made final decisions on diagnosis and treatment.[15] Additionally, unlike their male counterparts, the *ŭinyŏ* did not operate private practices but were dependent on the state medical institution to which they were assigned. The *Annals of the Chosŏn Dynasty* (*Chosŏn wangjo sillok*) recorded the names of renowned *ŭinyŏ* whose medical skills were rewarded with grains and release from their *ch'ŏnmin* status.[16]

It was due to prescribed gender customs that the *ŭinyŏ* were designated the *ch'ŏnmin* social status. The nature of their work demanded physical and social contact with male patients and bureaucrats, which did not make it possible for the *ŭinyŏ* to adhere to the principle of separation between males and females expected of higher status women. Ambiguity in terms of the *ŭinyŏ*'s function and place explains their association with state-regulated *kisaeng* female entertainers in the late nineteenth century.[17] Other nonmedical roles the *ŭinyŏ* may have been called upon to perform included inspection of wedding gifts and criminal investigations. The conflation of roles persisted throughout the dynasty and accounted for Horace Allen's frustrations with the female medical helpers assigned him by the court.

Scholars have noted a popularization of medicine beyond state medical institutions that occurred in Chosŏn in the eighteenth and nineteenth centuries with the emergence of an expanding market of *materia medica*, private practitioners, and publication of medical texts.[18] Other health providers included acupuncturists, tumor or abscess specialists, bonesetters, ritual healers and shamans, itinerant drug peddlers, smallpox inoculators (using the human variolation method), and local midwives who were not formally trained but were called on for their skills and experience.[19] The challenges posed by foreign settlements, rampant epidemics, and the closing of certain medical institutions in the late nineteenth century created opportunities for those existing practitioners who picked up new medical techniques and goods as they competed with new health workers.[20] Entrepreneurs sold foreign pharmaceutical goods and manufactured patent medicines or familiar herbal formulas packaged in new forms such as pills or powders.[21] Foreign-managed hospitals, dispensaries, and clinics employed Korean workers from across the social spectrum to assist in waiting rooms, pharmacies, wards, and consulting and surgical rooms. The modest medical training they offered set the stage for the growth of new medical professions.

In 1900, the Taehan state promulgated regulations to define the physician, pharmacist, and drug seller.[22] The new designation *ŭisa* for physician suggests a demarcation from earlier forms of elite medical practice enmeshed with Confucian state institutions, social status, and scholarship. Yet, as Soyoung Suh explains, the Chinese character *sa* (士; scholar) used then as a part of the translation for "physician," reflects the turn-of-the-twentieth-century image of physicians as Confucian scholarly gentlemen with a calling rather than skilled technicians or masters of biomedical knowledge. The definition of physician according to the regulation included "knowing the environmental cycle of Heaven and Earth, diagnosing the symptoms by pulse, and mastering (medical) classics and formulae," elements associated with Sino-classical medical traditions.[23] Qualifying for the Government Medical School required reading and composing in classical Chinese.[24] The majority of examinees at the medical qualifying exams administered in March 1900 were practitioners in the Sino-classical medical tradition.[25] Nevertheless, while new-style physicians were not easily rid of their former associations with classical scholarship, stipulations that licenses be awarded to graduates of proper medical colleges or pharmaceutical courses or to those who passed a state examination appear as attempts to standardize medical occupations along the lines of biomedicine.

As Korea became a protectorate and then a formal colony of Japan, the delineation between biomedicine and Sino-classical medicine became codified with the Regulation for Physicians promulgated by the GGK in 1913. While scholars have observed that it was not in the agenda of the GGK to provide a comprehensive medical system that addressed all health problems and offered Koreans full access to services, the GGK did seek a health administration that could effectively manage contagious diseases determined to be serious threats (such as cholera and smallpox), protect the health of its settler population, ameliorate relations with its colonized subjects (by offering free services in outpatient clinics), and allow Japan to boast in the international community that it was meeting its "civilizing" duty in its colony.[26] Doing so required the GGK to organize the piecemeal reforms and activities of foreign missionaries and the Taehan state to not only stipulate the education and activities of physicians but also construct a network of public hospitals as well as a sanitary administration run by a police bureaucracy that increasingly intervened in the colonized subjects' daily lives.

The 1913 Regulation for Physicians changed the Chinese character "*sa*" in *ŭisa* to a different Chinese character (師) with the same phonetic reading that meant "teacher." The title *ŭisa* was now reserved solely for those trained in and practicing biomedicine. It is also the term that is used today to translate physician into Korean. To qualify for a physician's license, one could produce certification from the Japanese government in Japan, graduate from a medical educational institution accredited by the GGK (usually a university medical school or four-year medical college), or pass a licensing examination based on biomedicine.[27] Graduating from an accredited medical school offered physicians a license to practice anywhere in Japanese territories, whereas those who qualified for a license by examination were limited to practice only in Korea. Initially, the only school in Korea that received this accreditation was the Medical Training Institute attached to the GGK Hospital (*Chosŏn ch'ongdokpu ŭiwŏn pusok ŭihak kangsŭpso*, hereafter GGK Hospital Training Institute). Some Koreans chose to study medicine abroad at accredited medical schools, principally in Japan, to receive the required qualification for a license upon graduation without having to take an examination.

To facilitate the transition to the new licensing system, some physicians who did not quite meet the standards as laid out by the Regulation for Physicians received a restricted license that was temporary and limited the spatial reach of the licensee's activity, usually to a rural or mountainous area in the provinces that lacked physicians. For the first few years after the promulgation of the Regulation for Physicians, foreign missionary physicians received this kind of license.[28] Ultimately, however, they too, like their Korean counterparts, had to pass the licensing exam or graduate from an accredited institution.[29] The strict standards set to receive a license account for the drastic drop in the number of licensed physicians from 1,712 in 1910 to 872 in 1915, according to GGK records.[30]

Furthermore, the Regulation for Physicians defined and monitored the activities of physicians.[31] If a physician had a private practice, s/he was required to report to the local police whenever opening, closing, or moving it. The Regulation authorized physicians to authenticate birth certificates and indicate the cause of death on death certificates, these too to be recorded with the police. It standardized procedures for filling out prescriptions and prohibited physicians from false advertising. Physicians became subject to malpractice suits if they abused their privileges. The Regulation did not, however, stipulate that the sex of a physician had to be male. In other words, women were not restricted from practicing medicine so long as they received the proper license. This was different from the regulations the GGK passed for nurses and midwives, discussed in a later chapter, which stated that these occupations were to be filled by women.

To meet the shortage of available Korean medical personnel trained in biomedicine, the GGK licensed a category of practitioners trained in Sino-classical medical traditions that became loosely categorized by various terms such as *hanbang* (Chinese medicine; J. *kanpō*), *tongŭi* (Eastern medicine), and *Chosŏnŭi* (Korean medicine). These practitioners were given the less prestigious appellation *ŭisaeng* (medical apprentices) according to the Regulation for *Ŭisaeng*, promulgated the same year as the Regulation for Physicians in 1913.[32] The *ŭisaeng* license was unique in the Japanese empire and represented a Japanese colonialist compromise: privileging biomedicine while allowing for the continuation of traditional Korean medicine.[33] To receive this license, one had to pass an examination that displayed a rudimentary knowledge of biomedical theories and techniques, particularly in the tenets of hygiene and disease prevention. *Ŭisaeng* organizations that emerged after 1913 published journals and texts aimed to provide this information to its members.[34]

The regulation, however, did not stipulate the kinds of treatment *ŭisaeng* could or could not practice. In fact, they too had the same authority to report birth or death certificates as did licensed physicians. Some *ŭisaeng* even found employment as public physicians (*kongŭi*) to work in sanitary administration with the police and in public hospitals in the provinces away from urban centers.[35] However, there was no doubt as to the status of *ŭisaeng* as second-tier practitioners: their license was limited to five years and depended on the needs and customs of Koreans.[36] Moreover, the GGK made no effort to provide any funds or support for the medical education of *ŭisaeng*. In the view of health administrators, they were to perform supportive roles in sanitary administration, especially in control measures against communicable diseases organized by the police, while curative services were reserved for licensed physicians.[37] Nevertheless, for most of the colonial period, the number of *ŭisaeng* outnumbered that of physicians.

CULTIVATING THE CLINICIAN

The professionalization of physicians rested on the foundation of new-style hospitals that trained and employed physicians and lay at the heart of medical services in Korea. As mentioned in the previous chapter, Japanese settlers established military hospitals and sanitation projects in treaty-port areas and the capital. Japanese physicians migrated to Korea in search of new opportunities, opening private practices and hospitals along the railroads in centers such as Taegu and Pyongyang and

TABLE 1.   Numbers of Licensed Physicians and *Ŭisaeng*

	1910	1915	1920	1925	1930	1935	1940
Physicians, Korean	1,342	209	402	637	921	1,336	1,918
Physicians, Japanese	345	627	604	685	796	1,146	1,269
Physicians, Foreign	25	36	29	36	32	24	10
Physicians, Total	1,712	872	1,035	1,358	1,749	2,506	3,197
Ŭisaeng	n/a	5,804	5,376	4,915	4,594	4,044	3,604

Source: *Chōsen sōtokofu tōkei nenpō* (various years).

participating in the administration of local hygiene work. Some Japanese Dōjinkai hospitals began offering medical education in 1907. The Pyongyang branch graduated its first class in 1910, the first time a Japanese-established medical educational institution graduated Korean students.[38] The Taehan state's Government Medical School graduated its first class in 1902.

Some Koreans received medical education in hospitals run by foreign missionaries such as the royal hospital Chejungwŏn—which was turned over to foreign mission boards in 1894 and renamed Severance Union Hospital—and East Gate Women's Hospital, their training programs being the predecessors to Yonsei University College of Medicine and Ewha Womans University College of Medicine, respectively. Severance graduated its first class of seven in 1908 but medical training at East Gate did not become institutionalized as an accredited medical school by the GGK during the colonial period.[39] In 1907, the Japanese RG constructed the Taehan Hospital, absorbing the Taehan state's hospital Kwangjewŏn and functions of the Korean Red Cross Hospital and vaccination centers.[40] The medical school affiliated with Taehan Hospital graduated fifty-four students in 1910, who then were appointed to positions in the Taehan Hospital, the RG's Bureau of Hygiene, or the military as army physicians.[41]

One of the first orders of business the GGK undertook upon colonizing Korea in 1910 was to expand a colony-wide system of public hospitals begun by the RG.[42] Over time, this was transformed from a series of primarily relief-providing charity hospitals (*chahye ŭiwŏn*), renamed provincial hospitals (*torip ŭiwŏn*) in 1925, into advanced educational and research facilities.[43] These regional hospitals were located in areas of political, military, and economic interest to the state, such as provincial capitals, major ports and railroad stations, and the border to the north. Other public hospitals included smaller-scale local hospitals at the municipal or district levels in Seoul, Pusan, Inch'ŏn, and the Hansen's disease (leprosy) asylum at Sorokdo (Deer Island), among others.[44]

At the apex of public hospitals after 1910 was the Taehan Hospital in the capital, now renamed the GGK Hospital.[45] Its affiliated medical school, the GGK Hospital Training Institute, sought to train Korean physicians, whose numbers were inadequate for the size of Korea's population.[46] However, the quality of education at the GGK Hospital Training

Institute was suspect at the beginning. Medical education in colonial Korea followed the same hierarchically tiered pyramid structure of general education as in Japan, with imperial universities (*cheguk taehak*) at the top, colleges or professional or specialized schools (*chŏnmun hakkyo*) below, followed by vocational or training institutes (*kangsŭpso*). Employment possibilities varied depending on the type of school one attended. As stipulated by the Regulation for Physicians, the kind of physician license for which one qualified depended on his/her education and if necessary, performance on a licensing examination. Moreover, public hospitals in Korea often preferred graduates from imperial universities with extra training in medical specialties. The student body of the GGK Hospital Training Institute was thus only Korean.[47] The lack of accreditation as a medical college that would grant a license to practice medicine upon graduation without additional qualification, as well as the lack of prestige, discouraged Japanese students from attending a school they perceived as inferior.[48]

The historiography of medical education in Korea debates whether the GGK's educational focus in Korea on basic literacy and technical skills and not on the production of a large class of highly educated professionals was intentional as a technique of colonial rule and discipline, a side effect of limited resources and time, or simply a structural consequence given the educational level of Koreans. On the one hand, the location of public hospitals suggests that the primary target of GGK medical administration was the Japanese settler population and that there was a reluctance to promote higher medical education for Koreans out of fear that Korean patients would become reliant on Korean and not Japanese physicians.[49] On the other hand, the GGK Hospital Training Institute stipulated that a prospective student had to know Japanese (the language of instruction) and have finished normal education at a time when education was a relatively new phenomenon and not a universal for Koreans, thus restricting the number who could even qualify to apply to the GGK Hospital Training Institute in the first place. As the normal school system provided schooling only until middle school (higher common) grades, the GGK Hospital Training Institute adopted teaching methods so students could learn medical techniques quickly and with relative ease; hence the curriculum's orientation toward clinical practice.[50] In any event, those who did manage to attend faced limited employment opportunities, with about a third of graduates from 1911–1915 choosing private practice while about half were employed in public hospitals as medical assistants and translators.[51]

The increasing prestige of the GGK Hospital Training Institute did confer some benefits even for Korean students. One promising development in 1914, for example, was a ruling that graduation from the GGK Hospital Training Institute automatically granted a license to practice medicine as a physician. No other medical training program in Korea, including the one at Severance, was allowed this privilege at that time. In 1916, the GGK Hospital Training Institute's status was upgraded to the level of professional school and renamed the Keijō Medical College (*Kyŏngsŏng ŭihak chŏnmun hakkyo*), becoming a choice destination for aspiring Japanese medical students. However, as in colonial Taiwan, it maintained its focus on producing clinicians rather than academics.[52] The GGK Hospital remained the site for the students' clinical education until 1928.

The difference in educational opportunities for Koreans and Japanese was manifested in structural inequalities. Japanese students who matriculated having achieved high school level education in Japan were granted a different status at Keijō Medical College and graduated with a special license that allowed them to practice in Japan as well. Korean graduates who entered Keijō Medical College with only four years of higher common (middle) school training received a license to practice limited to Korea. They did not receive a license that allowed them to practice in Japan until 1923, when education reforms extended common school education in Korea to match that in Japan.[53] Moreover, coursework differed for Japanese and Korean students. Korean students often organized to call for equal treatment, such as the same number of hours of instruction in mathematics and physics.[54] Since a major goal of the colonial authorities was to train Japanese physicians to fill positions at public hospitals in Korea, admission practices until 1922 specified that Japanese students comprise about one-third of the entering class, with the remaining two-thirds reserved for Korean students.[55] The number of Japanese students grew steadily from 1916, so that by 1924 they outnumbered Korean students.[56]

The priority of training academic Japanese physicians became even more pronounced with the establishment of Keijō Imperial University Medical Department (hereafter KIUMD) in 1926. GGK regulations for Keijō Medical College mandated that basic medical knowledge be learned through practice and discouraged a reliance on difficult German medical texts unless necessary when teaching, at a time when German medicine was associated with advanced medicine.[57] Regulations for the mission medical school at Severance stipulated that students be assigned to assist in surgery and treat patients directly on clinical rounds. This contrasts with KIUMD, the pinnacle of medical education in Korea, with its emphasis on research in its laboratories, a teaching institution with patients at its affiliated hospital (taking over the GGK Hospital from Keijō Medical College in 1928), and a doctoral program started in 1932.[58] KIUMD was the campus where students were to learn the "theory and application of scholarship in demand by the state."[59] Students were expected to pursue research to advance medical knowledge. So, rather than focusing their classes on clinical lectures and practice as at the colleges, KIUMD students learned in laboratories and participated in various research institutions affiliated with the school.

Although KIUMD was located in Seoul, Korean students faced obstacles to study or work there. Following the system of imperial universities in Japan, KIUMD employed only Japanese nationals as full-time faculty or administrative officials. Throughout its twenty years, only two Koreans worked as assistant professors (one for thirteen months, the other for only three days), with a handful of Koreans serving as temporary assistants. Korean students made up less than 30 percent of total graduates.[60] While graduation from such an elite university should have opened more opportunities for Koreans, nearly half of the graduates from 1930 to 1941 opened their own practices, finding other avenues for employment limited.[61] On the one hand, private practice may have been more attractive to Koreans since it meant not having to face discriminatory practices in Japanese-administered hospitals. On the other hand, the road was tougher, with fewer resources and facilities. Setting up a private practice was costly—physicians had to cover rent, pay any staff they hired, and purchase medical supplies and medications to use in their practice.[62] Moreover, they had no privileges at hospitals so could not continue treating patients they sent to be hospitalized.[63]

Although what emerged for the medical profession in colonial Korea was a Japanese empire–oriented education and training system that entailed marginalization of Korean medical students and practitioners, there nonetheless were employment opportunities to fill gaps in the Japanese-dominated system.[64] The public hospitals tended to hire Japanese physicians over Koreans. As Pak Yunjae notes, if Korean physicians were so fortunate as to be hired at a public hospital, they usually took "leftover" positions.[65] Or they were hired in the welfare department of the hospital that handled the dispensary or charity outpatient work with Korean patients.[66] Private hospitals, while not under the direct administration of the GGK except in terms of registration, consisted primarily of clinics, dispensaries, and mission hospitals and offered a few additional opportunities for Korean physicians.[67] Another option for Korean physicians was employment with the sanitary police as public physicians, medical officers who were under the jurisdiction of the police, but also were allowed to maintain private practices so long as those did not interfere with their sanitary administrative duties.[68] Intended initially to address the health needs of Japanese residents, the first public physicians were Japanese. However, the inferior conditions and status of public physicians, when a graduate from a recognized medical school could earn more with a private practice in an urban area, and the fact that academic medicine was considered more prestigious than public health administration, meant that there were insufficient numbers of Japanese physicians. Korean physicians thus became employable as public physicians.

New opportunities in medical education formed the basis for the growth of a new medical professional class. Despite the initial decline of licensed physicians with the 1913 Regulation for Physicians, Korean physicians grew steadily in number, wealth, and prestige in stark contrast to medical missionary Oliver R. Avison's 1893 observation that men from *yangban* elite status found the work of physicians abhorrent due to its connotations of *chungin* secondary status and physical contact with diseased or injured bodies.[69] As tuition at Keijō Medical College and Severance amounted to roughly two thousand yen (at a time when one would need fifty yen a month to live comfortably), attending medical school was possible for only the wealthy.[70] But those who could afford it also expected to receive a return on their investment. Physicians were among the best-paid professionals in this period, earning around one hundred yen a month, more than three hundred yen with a successful practice. The respectability of science, which was presented as the foundation of medical practice, provided physicians a further boost in prestige, even while complaints were levied against physicians who were likened to "thieves" for overcharging for the medications they prescribed their patients.[71] Another attraction was that medicine was considered a stable occupation.

Physicians penned editorials and columns on health issues in popular print media and participated in civic organizations.[72] In 1915, Korean physicians organized the Seoul Association of Physicians (*Hansŏng ŭisahakhoe*, 1915–1941) as a networking organization for physicians in Seoul, a conscious counterpart to the Korean Medical Association (*Chosŏn ŭihakhoe*, 1911–1943), the professional organization of Japanese physicians in Korea.[73] The Seoul Association of Physicians engaged in medical volunteer and sanitary activities and organized themselves to promote what they perceived to be Korea's health interests, demanding, for example, a thorough investigation of and compensation for the untimely deaths of Koreans given emetine injections in 1927.[74] Other areas, such as Pyongyang, established local physician associations as well. In 1930, Korean physicians organized the Association of Korean Physicians (*Chosŏn ŭisa hyŏphoe*) with a focus on the publication of medical research. Partly in response to Japanese research on racial biometrics, they published in the Association's journal, *Chosŏn ŭibo* (1930–1937), medical research conducted by Korean physicians.[75] Korean physicians also endeavored to differentiate themselves from and discredit traditional Korean medical practices by engaging in a very public and long series of debates with *hanbang* medical practitioners in the 1930s.

Despite the difficulties, the model of a patronage system that Byonghee Cho uses to explain the relationship between the colonial state and physicians accounts for why Korean physicians shared the same values as the colonial state on matters of public health and medicine.[76] The GGK monopolized education, employment practices, and hospital services through its network of public hospitals. The state was the major employer of physicians and held the choicest positions, which for the most part were not available to Korean physicians. Physicians outside the public hospital system—in private practice or mission hospitals—faced tough competition as the reputation, prestige, and facilities of public hospitals surpassed others in the eyes of the populace.[77] This produced a pressure or tendency for Korean physicians to adopt the values, practices, and attitudes of physicians in public hospitals that was difficult to overcome. Female physicians found themselves dealing with not only gender practices but also the structural inequalities embedded in the colonial administration of medicine.

MAKING A CASE FOR THE FEMALE PHYSICIAN

In 1909, the bulletin of the academic society Taehan Hŭnghakhoe published a forceful call for women to study medicine. In these revolutionary times, the author asserted, female students should break forth from their former lives of seclusion in the inner quarters. How could they yield the responsibilities of learning and representing the country's women to men alone?[78] To potential skeptics, the author argued that the development of women's skills and education was necessary for them to perform the duties of the Wise Mother, Good Wife and establish proper homes. The area of most urgency was medicine. It was a contradiction that the field be historically dominated by men when the *naewoebŏp* (inner/outer principle) separation between sexes restricted men so that even at their patients' sickbeds they could do no more than diagnose through checking of the *maek* (meridian channels).[79] The author, moreover, was skeptical of Sino-classical medical traditions that purported to treat all the myriad complaints women suffered. While both men and women experienced colds, "cold damage" disorders, fevers, and aches, women also were afflicted with ailments specific to women. Their reluctance to show their bodies to either their mother or father, much less a male physician, could lead to misdiagnosis or delayed treatment.

This piece articulated four concerns about the general situation of females that repeatedly emerged in discussions about female medical training and professionalization in the early twentieth century. First, due to the customary separation of the sexes, female patients were reluctant to see male physicians. Women's hesitance also may have been due, in part, to the general embarrassment female patients felt when examined. This likely arose from the second concern, the gender-specific ailments women suffered, as the ailments the author lists—uterine disease (*cha-gung pyŏng*), "symptoms below the waist" (*taehajŭng*), and irregular menstrual cycles—all relate to the female reproductive system. That women would resist such intimate physical examinations is buttressed by the reactions of even lower-status women to examinations for venereal disease made compulsory by a new system of licensed prostitution.[80]

Focus on the gynecological concerns of women raises the third concern: the article's implicit critique of *hanbang* methods and folk healing techniques that many female patients continued to utilize, particularly when addressing what was understood as female complaints. The author's final concern relates to the higher education of women. Medicine, as an ideal profession for women because their knowledge of and participation in health activities directly related to their performance of ideal womanhood and proper domesticity, required more formal education and training than most occupations women pursued in colonial Korea.

The colonial government's administration of Korea's public health and medical infrastructure only reinforced these concerns. Goals for female education and medicine converged most poignantly on the issue of maternal and infant health. In 1915, a Japanese midwife contributed an article to the colonialist journal *Chōsen oyobi Manshu* (Korea and Manchuria) that shocked its readers with "the horror suffered by unfortunate Korean women during labor on account of their superstition, the primitive knowledge of sanitation possessed by them and their relatives, and their dislike of being attended by male physicians."[81] Many women died prematurely due to their refusal to see a male physician when sick or in labor, and, although foreign missionaries and the GGK put effort into training nurses and midwives, it was not enough. Thus, the author pressed for the means to produce "as many well-trained midwives, nurses, and female physicians as possible in the shortest possible time." "In fact," she continued, "in no other country in the Far East is the need of training and educating women as physicians and midwives greater."[82] While, admittedly, there was yet no medical school for women in Korea, she hoped that "private and Government or public higher schools for Korean girls, will encourage students having a liking for natural sciences to qualify themselves for medicine."

Gendered protocols in social interactions and the valorization of prescribed care-providing roles permitted medicine to become one of the respectable occupations available to women. Yet the strict requirements and structural inequalities in medical schools that restricted offerings available to Korean men hindered Korean women even more. It took formidable strength, resources, and perhaps luck for a woman in this period to receive a medical education, much less a medical license and the opportunity to practice. On principle, neither public nor mission medical schools accepted women as students, apart from a few women auditors at the GGK Hospital Training Institute discussed further below. Excluded from conventional routes to medicine available to men in Korea, early female physicians had to seek alternate means to receive a medical education.

The first Korean woman to receive a medical degree was Esther Pak (née Kim Chŏmdong) whose Christian family background placed her in contact with missionaries and their institutions.[83] Initially recruited to translate for Dr. Rosetta S. Hall at the mission women's hospital Pogunyŏgwan, Pak soon began to assist Hall in the dispensary and hospital as her interest in medicine deepened. She accompanied Hall and her children to the United States to study medicine when Hall went on furlough in 1896. There, Pak studied English and nursing in New York before entering the Women's Medical College in Baltimore, from which she received her medical degree in 1900. Like her Chinese counterparts returning to China, Pak was appointed a missionary to Korea by the WFMS.[84] She worked in Seoul at Pogunyŏgwan upon her return to Korea before moving to Pyongyang in 1903 to work with Dr. Hall at the mission's Kwanghye Women's Hospital there. Dedicated to the medical care of women and children, Pak worked tirelessly before succumbing to tuberculosis in 1910. It was her life that inspired Dr. Hall's son, Sherwood Hall, to later pursue a medical degree to specialize in tuberculosis work as a missionary in Korea.[85]

Mission reports indicate that another Korean woman, recorded by her English name Grace Lee, was the first Korean woman to receive a medical-related license from the GGK.[86] Trained as a nurse in mission hospitals Grace was representative of the kinds of women of marginal status initially recruited for mission nursing training programs. She was of the lowest *ch'ŏnmin* status. Her involvement in medicine began when she approached missionaries to relieve her suffering from an affliction that required the removal of a necrotic bone.[87] Likely because her medical training did not meet the physician *ŭisa* licensing standards set by the GGK, Lee was granted a *ŭisaeng* license in 1914. Another Korean woman in Pyongyang also received a *ŭisaeng* license although it is not clear if she, like Grace Lee, had a nursing background before practicing medicine.[88]

There was just too little opportunity for women to study medicine in Korea, much less receive higher education.[89] Until a medical school for women opened in Korea in 1928, women's only recourse was to study abroad or privately (for example, work with missionaries such as Rosetta S. Hall and Mary Cutler at East Gate Women's Hospital in Seoul and Kwanghye Women's Hospital in Pyongyang) and pass the licensing exam.[90] From its opening in 1928, the Korean Women's Medical Training Institute (hereafter, Training Institute) was considered subpar, not upgraded to professional school status until 1938. The other medical schools available in the 1920s—Severance, Keijō Professional Medical School, KIUMD, and later the training departments at the provincial hospitals in Taegu and Pyongyang—did not accept women as students. The only notable exception was made in 1916 when missionaries negotiated with the GGK Hospital Training Institute School to accept five of their students as auditors. Three of the five students—An Sugyŏng, Kim Haeji (Hattie Kim), and Kim Yŏnghŭng—graduated in 1918 and were granted licenses to practice without further examination.[91] Upon these female students' graduation, Governor-General Terauchi commended them for "they will undoubtedly not spare their noble effort for Korean women and children."[92] He hoped that other women would follow their example.

During their medical training at the GGK Hospital Training Institute (later Keijō Medical College), these female students sat separately from the male students and lived in a separate dormitory with supervision. Although their tuition was waived, they had to work seven to nine hours a day, six days a week, in the hospital's scullery, laundry, pharmacy, or dispensary.[93] They boarded and cooked for themselves at their own expense. The female students also had to be accompanied by chaperones to their classrooms. Receiving instructions in the Japanese language was decidedly difficult for them considering that their initial medical instructions with missionaries had been in English.[94] One of the five quit medical studies apparently because of difficulty with the Japanese language, while another decided she would rather study medicine in the United States. The Keijō Medical College continued to accept female auditors until 1923.[95] One observer speculated in 1927 that this may have been because authorities were not pleased with the results or because it was deemed that there were too many embarrassing subjects in physiology and hygiene for female students to study alongside male students.[96] An estimated seven to eight female physicians were trained in this way.[97]

In fact, contact with missionaries through their schools or hospitals was the main way a woman could study medicine in the early years of Japanese colonial rule. Rosetta S. Hall noted there were twelve Korean female physicians in 1925, and, of these, only two had pursued medical education or employment that had no association with missionaries.[98] The rest either began their medical studies in mission hospitals in Korea or China (Union Women's Medical College in Beijing), or if they received a degree from Tokyo Women's Medical College, found employment in mission institutions upon receiving a license to practice.[99] For example, Tokyo Women's Medical College graduates Chŏng Chayŏng, Hyŏn Tŏksin, and Kil Chŏnghŭi worked at East Gate Women's Hospital.[100] Among the twelve listed by Hall was Song Poksin, who received the Barbour scholarship for Asian women at the University of Michigan and expected to work at a mission hospital upon her return.[101] She was the first Korean woman to receive a medical PhD in 1929, but decided not to return to Korea after marrying an American.[102]

The medical education of women had long been an area of interest to missionaries. Rosetta S. Hall noted the saying "It is as natural for a woman to be a doctor as to be a mother" and advised that "the quality of children rather than their quantity be better considered."[103] Yet, as she quoted an observer from the Methodist General Board, the need for medical work "*for women by women* in Korea was *not* being met by the Government hospitals or private doctors."[104] This was a "gross neglect" of women and children. Training women was not about taking work away from men, she claimed, for midwifery was women's God-given task. An advocate for the health and welfare of women, children, and the deaf and blind, Hall made it her main ambition to establish a medical school for women in Korea.

Her efforts to start a Korean medical school for women was realized when she joined forces with physicians Kil Chŏnghŭi, who had graduated from Tokyo Women's Medical College (the premier medical educational institution for women in the Japanese empire) in 1923, and her husband Kim Tagwŏn, a graduate of Keijō Medical College and later president of the Seoul Association of Physicians. In 1928, the Training Institute began with volunteer instructors and fifteen students, five of whom constituted its first graduating class in 1934.[105] All apparently received their medical licenses after passing the GGK-administered examination. The school graduated its second class of five in 1936.[106] Its dependence on mission support, however, undermined its ability to survive. Rosetta S. Hall lobbied mission boards, secured scholarship funds from the Women's Medical Society of New York, and used her personal connections to secure the site (home of her friend and fellow missionary), and faculty for the Training Institute. This, however, left the school on shaky ground when Hall retired in 1933. The Training Institute had to vacate its building, as it was considered property of the mission, and lost financial support from the American mission community.[107]

With the removal of its association with missionaries, the Training Institute changed its name in 1933 to Keijō Women's Medical Training Institute at the behest of the GGK.[108] Under the leadership of the husband-wife team of Kim Tagwŏn and Kil Chŏnghŭi, the Training Institute established a school association (*Kyo'uhoe*) to build collegiality and share news and medical knowledge among its membership of present and former faculty, staff, students, and honorary members.[109] The association published the inaugural issue of its bulletin *Kyo'u hoeji* in 1934 and mobilized influential members of Korean society to promote legal recognition of the Training Institute as a professional school.[110] Yet the GGK remained indifferent to the Training Institute's difficulties, much to Kil's chagrin. As she later recalled in her memoir, the GGK would not support women's medical education unless the school raised ten million yen in private funds.[111] Thanks to the donation of Korean philanthropist Kim Chong'ik upon his death in 1937 the school did acquire the funds necessary to upgrade to professional school status and gain recognition by the GGK as Keijō Women's Medical College in 1938.

With its professional school status, the number of enrolled students, including Japanese, jumped significantly. The GGK, pleased with the increase in the number of students at the new school, also began to make annual contributions. The Keijō Women's Medical College graduated its first class of 47 students (4 of them Japanese) in 1942.[112] By the time Japan's colonial rule ended in Korea in 1945, there were some 200 Korean women enrolled at Keijō Women's Medical College.

Other students seeking medical education elected to study abroad, particularly in Japan. The majority of those who studied in Japan attended Tokyo Women's Medical College while others attended the Teikoku Women's Medical College (est. 1925) or Osaka Women's Higher Medical College (est. 1928).[113] About a hundred Korean women studied medicine in Japan during the colonial period, making up about 13 percent of the total number of Korean female students who studied in Japan.[114] The first Korean woman to receive her medical degree there was Hŏ Yŏngsuk, the wife of the famed and controversial literary figure Yi Kwangsu. Hŏ graduated from Tokyo Women's Medical College in 1917 and became the first Korean woman to receive the medical *ŭisa* license after the 1913 Regulation for Physicians was enacted. A few students with mission connections attended the Union Medical College in Beijing or went to the United States, but studying abroad was no easy task. Kil Chŏnghŭi remembers how sad she felt about leaving home but dared not disobey her grandfather's wish that she study medicine. There were three Koreans in her class at Tokyo Women's Medical College. They were behind in language and so had lower grades than their Japanese classmates, who lent them notes to study with as they worked hard to keep up with their coursework. The friendship Kil felt for her Japanese classmates, however, was sorely tested during the anti-Korean attacks in the aftermath of the 1923 Kantō earthquake.[115]

A DOUBLE-EDGED SWORD

Even when fortunate enough to receive a medical education and a physician's license, a woman faced ambivalence from patients, family, and colleagues toward her participation in medicine. Women were generally excluded from professional associations. The first female member of the

Seoul Association of Physicians was Chŏng Chayŏng in 1938, after she had been practicing medicine since graduating from Tokyo Women's Medical College two decades earlier in 1918.[116] What makes this late inclusion of women even more strange is the fact that a major member, and even president (1931–1932) of the Seoul Association of Physicians was Kim Tagwŏn, the dean of the Training Institute after Rosetta S. Hall's retirement, and a strong supporter of the education and activities of female physicians. Nor did Korean female physicians themselves organize their own professional organization, although many of them were involved in other women's and student organizations.[117] This could be due to their small numbers or the fact that physician associations in Korea at that time were centered around either publication of advanced medical research, for which few female physicians had the credentials, or fraternizing. Moreover, the Training Institute's association *Kyo'u hoe* was dominated by male physicians as it organized around the cause of upgrading the Training Institute to a professional school.

Unfortunately, there are no official statistics on female physicians from this period. Colonial authorities conscientiously tabulated collected data on the population based on different categories, such as birth, marriage, and occupation. These figures were then broken down further into detailed configurations such as sex, nationality, age, month, and region.[118] Physicians, however, were categorized only by the type of license they had (*ŭisa*, *ŭisaeng*, "restricted" *ŭisa*) and nationality. This may reflect the fact that generally Korean physicians were male. If Rosetta S. Hall's 1925 estimate was accurate, then there were only twelve female physicians out of a total of 637 Korean physicians recorded by the GGK. These twelve included Esther Pak, by then deceased, and two who received a *ŭisaeng* license.[119] Growth in female physicians was decidedly slow. A decade later, female physicians numbered somewhere between thirty and fifty. Female physicians themselves were unsure of their own numbers as they had no professional organization. At a 1934 round-table discussion of female physicians published in the women's journal *Sin kajŏng*, Chang Mungyŏng guessed their number to be around fifty while Ryu Yŏngjun thought thirty.[120] In 1935, female physician Son Ch'ijŏng estimated a total of forty female physicians in Korea.[121] The Training Institute's association *Kyo'u hoe* listed fourteen female physicians, five alums, and forty-one current students among its members in

1934.[122] Other members included the school's faculty, staff, honorary members, and those who contributed to the establishment or operation of the Training Institute.

Despite the earnest efforts to broaden opportunities for women to become physicians, the reality was that not many women chose medicine as a career path. Those who did faced many hurdles, often dropping out of medical studies or practice. Finances, of course, were an issue. Female physician Son Ch'ijŏng noted how the depressed economic situation in the 1930s made it even more difficult to send women abroad for study.[123] Rosetta S. Hall complained that mission support of $150 per student was needed for their study abroad. And by 1930, the GGK no longer offered financial support for students seeking to study medicine in Japan. Thus, the majority of women who studied medicine abroad came from families with the means and will to support their education. Moreover, despite the relatively high income expected from public hospital employment, female physicians had an even more difficult time than their male counterparts in finding such employment. While a few female physicians did find employment at large hospitals, these positions tended to be temporary.[124] A 1927 *Pyŏlgŏngon* article concluded that, in general, female physicians overall did not earn much despite the claim laid out at the beginning of this chapter. If they did, one observer asked, why would so few open private practices and leave so soon?[125] One physician recalled how difficult it was to maintain a lucrative private practice; she often, for example, received no payment for attending deliveries.[126]

Other students bowed to the family pressures of marriage given the demands of the profession.[127] Medical work required much mental effort and stamina. Physicians worked late hours on occasion, making patient rounds, even visiting patients in their homes, all of which was physically taxing.[128] These duties were difficult to juggle with domestic tasks. Hŏ Yŏngsuk, for example, ended her private practice after only a few years for reasons, she suggested, that included caring for her family.[129] The wife of pediatrician Yi Sŏngŭn studied medicine in Japan and worked as a pediatrician at the GGK Hospital affiliated with KIUMD before quitting formal work to raise five children.[130] Even Kil Chŏnghŭi admitted in her memoir that she was only able to devote herself to her practice and the Training Institute because she did not have children immediately after her marriage.

The length of training was one of the reasons for this delay: upon graduation, a female physician usually had to work at least three years in a hospital or with a well-known physician to build experience and gain recognition. Kil, for example, postponed her work with the Training Institute because she wanted to pursue internships at the GGK Hospital and East Gate Women's Hospital before joining her husband's private practice. She worked there until Rosetta S. Hall's retirement in 1933 prompted her return to become assistant principal at the Training Institute. Her experience also illustrates how medicine as a profession could postpone marriage for women. She remarked that the newspapers called her an "old maid" when she married at age twenty-six.

Other challenges faced women as physicians. They were discouraged from pursuing medical specialties other than gynecology and pediatrics. In the inaugural issue of *Kyo'u hoeji*, all three of the academic treatises published were related to those two fields—mental health and its effect on women's reproductive system, menses and pregnancy, and family medicine with its focus on pediatrics, the lectures of the second series of public health lectures given by the school's faculty and students in 1933. The first series of lectures also focused on women's reproductive health and the digestive ailments of children.[131] As one female physician who graduated from the Keijō Women's Medical College later explained, she went into obstetrics-gynecology because, as a woman, she could not choose any other specialty.[132] Kil Chŏnghŭi recorded that few people were aware of female physicians. Her pride and confidence were challenged by her encounters with patients who assumed she was a midwife and not a physician. Moreover, despite their skills, female physicians often lacked credibility as physicians due to their sex. One commentator noted that female physicians such as Hŏ Yŏngsuk, Hyŏn Tŏksin, and Yi Tŏgyo were known more for their marriages to literary husbands than their medical expertise, even though Hŏ ran her own practice and Yi was temporarily employed by the GGK Hospital.[133] The anonymity of the aforementioned wife of pediatrician Yi Sŏngŭn in an article in a women's journal that featured their family and model relationship as a physician couple highlights the general marginalization of women in the medical profession, although she had once been employed at one of the most elite hospitals of the colonial period.[134] Hŏ Yŏngsuk found her skills as a physician undermined by even her own husband, Yi Kwangsu, who sought second opinions about medications she prescribed for their children when they were ill.[135] If the second opinion agreed with hers, Yi remained silent. However, if the prescriptions differed, he returned home to scold her.

Female physicians at the 1934 roundtable discussed above shared the numerous challenges and barriers they faced because of their sex and/or ethnicity. Ryu Yŏngjun recalled in dismay how she was called in the middle of the night to deliver a baby only to be unwelcomed, unappreciated, and unpaid for her efforts when her clients realized she was Korean. Another physician spoke about the hostile environment in medical education created by their male peers in Korea, and Ryu recounted the degrading treatment she and female physicians in general received in hospitals, not being recognized as physicians in their own right by their peers and patients but treated as nurses. They were assumed able to treat only female patients. Medicine was obviously not an occupation for the fainthearted.

Nevertheless, while it was not a common profession for Korean women, so long as one had the finances, will, and stamina to attend and graduate from an accredited medical school and/or pass the government licensing exam, becoming a physician was one of the few respectable and elite professions a woman could practice with a relatively high income and status. A woman physician could earn an initial salary of seventy to eighty yen in 1927, whereas an ordinary teacher and midwife could expect an initial salary of forty to fifty yen. Female radio announcers earned fifty to sixty yen, a top-earning female reporter received sixty to seventy yen, while nurses and telephone operators earned on the lower end of the scale (average thirty yen).[136] Kil Chŏnghŭi said she earned one hundred yen a month when working at the GGK and East Gate Women's Hospital. Unlike schoolteachers, female physicians could work from home if they opened up their own practices, though those could be difficult to maintain when patients declined to pay.

While the assumption that female physicians could treat only female patients may have been demoralizing, female physicians nonetheless did feel that they performed a much-needed service for which they as women were better suited and thus saw themselves as pioneers, contributing to the betterment of their communities. Female physicians themselves, for the most part, repeated similar gendered arguments for their participation as did missionaries and the 1909 observer in the Tae-han Hŭnghakhoe bulletin mentioned earlier. For example, Pak Sunjŏng, of the first graduating class, stated in the public lecture on family health that she contributed to the *Kyo'u hoeji*, "Women more than men need [medical] common knowledge" for they not only cook at home, which provides the basic nutrition humans need to survive, but also because it is women who raise children and thus carry the "large responsibil-ity of preserving the life of the race (*chongjok*)."[137] This resonates with the gendered citizenship discussed in the last chapter that informed much of the *wisaeng* instructions in schools and print media. Train-ing Institute student Chŏng Nami concurred that, in particular, it was more imperative for women than men to learn medical knowledge. "The improvement of human lifestyle by keeping our bodies healthy" starts with the family, then society, and only then will there be happiness in the whole country. This was the "important responsibility that women cannot avoid in their 'heavenly-task' (*ch'ŏnjik*) as mothers and masters of a household." The responsibility for the health of the country should not rest on only a few physicians, however, and thus Chŏng urged sup-port for recognition of the Training Institute as a professional school to further improve health in the home.[138]

Tokyo Women's Medical College graduate Ryu Yŏngjun further stressed the need for female physicians as it was mothers who were best able to deal with the health needs and welfare of their children "as only women know women's troubles best."[139] To the first graduat-ing class of the Training Institute she offered reaffirmation of their value as female physicians: "We women are tasked with the health of our families, raising of the next generation of citizens (*kungmin*), and taking one step further the health of our nation (*minjok*) and improve-ment of the race (*injong*)." Moreover, female physicians did not limit the scope of their responsibility to the provision of health instructions to housewives. They took pride in saving valuable lives in ways that their male colleagues could not. Ryu's fellow alum Hyŏn Tŏksin stressed the urgency for separate women's hospitals run by women to save women's lives because women at large not only did not have modern medical knowledge but also resisted visiting medical facilities with male patients and physicians.[140] Kil Chŏnghŭi admitted that her interest in medicine was on the orders of her grandfather, who saw women's participation in medicine as addressing the plight of female patients who received incorrect diagnoses and unnecessarily difficult labor that led occasionally to untimely deaths as they avoided male physicians.[141] She realized over time that to be responsible for the life of another was to do great things. Therefore, she believed she and others like her served a large purpose: the health of the family and society depended on the popularization and increasing acceptance of female physicians.[142] Female physicians were needed to help construct a new society.

CHAPTER 3

The Heavenly Task of Nursing

On January 22, 1924, the daily newspaper *Tonga ilbo* reported the formation of a new nursing association, the Korean Nurses' Society (*Chosŏn kanhobu hyŏphoe*; hereafter Nurses' Society). Two of the founding members were prominent Korean nurse-midwives, Han Singwang and Chŏng Chongmyŏng. As Han explained at the inaugural meeting attended by around thirty members, they were starting the Nurses' Society because "although the figure of the nurse in Korea had been around for a while, there was yet little activity among nurses to promote the nursing profession."[1] A few days after the announcement about the Nurses' Society, the *Tonga ilbo* published a photo of Han with American missionary and trained nurse Elma T. Rosenberger in an article about the new infant welfare work starting at T'aehwa Yŏjagwan (hereafter T'aehwa).[2] T'aehwa, called the Social Evangelistic Center by affiliated foreign missionaries, was a community center for Korean women and children founded in 1921 by the WFMS and the Women's Council of the Southern Methodist Church for evangelistic, educational, and social service purposes.[3] By the 1930s, T'aehwa was the center of mission infant welfare efforts.

Han Singwang was Rosenberger's assistant at T'aehwa's infant welfare clinic. Born into a Christian family in Kyŏngsang Province in 1902, Han attended Christian schools and taught kindergarten and elementary school before moving to Seoul in 1919 to enter the nursing training school at East Gate Women's Hospital, from which she graduated in spring 1923.[4] While a student, she did additional coursework in midwifery to prepare for the midwifery licensing exam, which she passed in June 1923. She was at that time one of only forty-two licensed Korean midwives in the country.[5] That Han Singwang was involved simultaneously with the work at T'aehwa and the new Nurses' Society is not surprising. What is surprising is the fact that Han helped organize the Nurses' Society at the same time she was actively involved with another nursing organization, the Korean Nurses' Association (*Chosŏn kanhobuhoe*; hereafter KNA). The KNA was closely associated with the foreign mission nursing community with which Han was professionally aligned. What was to be gained by starting another nursing organization when her work affiliation already linked her to mission medical work and the KNA?

This chapter addresses that question by examining the participation of missionaries in the professionalization of nursing and midwifery, which did not exist as formal occupations before the modern period. Caught within the boundaries set by the Japanese colonial state yet imbued by the mission to which they felt called, missionaries established nursing and midwifery training programs and waged public health campaigns. The relationship missionaries had with Korean health workers, patients, and Japanese authorities were at times receptive and collegial, at other times fraught with tension. Nonetheless, as the case of mission infant welfare programs demonstrates, missionaries opened new opportunities for women and laid the foundation for Korean female leadership in professional medical, public health, and social services.

FEMINIZING THE NURSE

The profession of nursing, like that of physician, developed in the context of the establishment of hospitals, clinics, and dispensaries in Korea under the increasing influence of medical practices of the West and Japan. The corralling of the sick and injured into hospital settings was new to Koreans—that families would send their loved ones away from their homes was difficult for them to comprehend at first. They resisted leaving the full-time care of family members to strangers at all, much less overnight in hospitals. Moreover, they found distasteful the foods offered, certain treatments associated with hospitals such as surgery, and hospital routines. Integral to the operation of the new hospitals were nurses who assisted physicians and attended to the ill. The first formal nursing training programs for Koreans began in foreign mission hospitals—the first students being hospital helpers and assistants in the dispensary at East

Gate Women's Hospital (1903) and Severance Hospital (1906)—before spreading to mission hospitals throughout the country.[6] Although mission hospitals found it necessary to train male nurses, it was expected that with the conversion and training of more Korean women, nurses eventually would all be female.[7] In 1907, two women graduated from their training to be the first capped Korean nurses.[8] Five more graduated the following year.[9] In 1909, at Severance, there were a total of ten nursing students.[10] Japanese hospitals too began nurse training programs before 1910, but these were geared primarily toward Japanese students. Dōjinkai hospitals began to train nurses in Pyongyang (1906) and Taegu (1907). The nurse training program at the Taehan Hospital was begun in 1908, but its Korean students were trained as *kyŏnsŭpsaeng*, or apprentices, in contrast to Japanese students, whose coursework put them on a path toward graduation.[11]

Initially, the assumption that nursing was a female vocation, premised on assertions of women's "motherly" or feminine nature, was not quite so evident as one might assume. As discussed in earlier chapters, providing medical care and nurturing the ill at home during the Chosŏn period was not necessarily associated with feminine traits nor were these tasks restricted to women. Elite Korean men considered medical knowledge in the Sino-classical tradition as part of their erudition and regarded the performance of informal medical care at home as fulfilling the Confucian virtue of filiality. *Yangban* household records, for example, show that men bought medicinal ingredients from the market to store at home and use to concoct medicines based on physicians' prescriptions or their own.[12] They also recorded the progress of illnesses within the family.

Moreover, that women as care providers and, by extension, nurses was not a "natural" concept is reflected in the evolution of the translation into Korean of the English term "nurse." During the cholera epidemic of 1895, the Korean government established temporary isolation hospitals in cooperation with foreign medical personnel, utilizing public health practices of the West to quickly detect and quarantine infected persons and thereby limit the extent of the contagion. The state hired temporary nurses, paying their wages as a sundry expense out of a separate budget from that for other medical personnel.[13] These early nurses were called *kanhobu* (man who watches over, protects, and aids), using the male Chinese character for *pu* (夫) instead of the female character *pu* (婦), for they were not female but male. The hospitals also received aid from a broad category of care providers called *kangbyŏngin* (person who watches over the ill) who were patients' family members or individuals hired privately by patients. Missionaries decided to translate nurse as *kanhowŏn* using the Chinese character *wŏn*, a gender-neutral appellation for "personnel," instead of the male *pu*.[14]

In their memoirs, missionaries observed that before formal programs for the training of Korean nurses began, medical institutions employed male medical assistants to care for male patients in medical facilities such as Chejungwŏn. The informal nursing staff at the isolation hospital put under the charge of missionary Lillias Underwood (née Horton) consisted of both men and women without concern for their traditional status.[15] The Korean Red Cross Hospital had two categories of nurses— *kanhojol* (army nurse), which reflected the military aspect of Japanese and Red Cross nursing, and *kanhobu* (with female *pu*), introducing the term that became the designation for nurse in colonial Korea.[16] The latter suggests that the term for nurse had begun to shift toward the feminine even though nurses were not necessarily female and the hospital appointed male officers in nursing administration.[17] According to a 1906 mission report, even missionaries at Severance Hospital hired male nurses.[18] That men served as nurses in this early period is evident in the fact that Korean female nurses did not nurse male patients until necessitated in 1907 by a nursing shortage brought about by a surge in the number of injured in the aftermath of the dispersal of the Korean army and subsequent increase in skirmishes with the Japanese military. Severance Hospital mobilized female nursing students from its training institute as well as from East Gate Women's Hospital, introducing female nurses slowly to work in male wards.[19] Even in the late 1920s, nursing was not a popular occupation for women in Hamhŭng Province in the north. Nurses in mission hospitals there tended to be male.[20]

Nevertheless, as nursing education and practice became systematized, it was clear that nursing was intended as a female profession. While missionaries may have employed male nurses, their ideal nurse was a woman of strong Christian faith. From the start of missionary nursing education, the female nurse was to be the "best embodiment [of] consecrated womanhood," as one missionary put it.[21] The Korean woman would make a good nurse, one commentator averred, for she is "naturally sympathetic, large hearted, and hospitable . . . wonderfully skilled in the use of her fingers and handles a cambric needle or a bandage with an exactness which is most pleasing."[22] While their duties were primarily to assist physicians, nurses also performed housekeeping duties such as sewing bed linens and hospital gowns, preparing and serving meals, and even cleaning or caring for corpses.[23] Nurses had to learn "obedience, patience, and gentleness," qualities that were not correspondingly demanded of male medical students.[24] They were trained in their duty to God, country, doctors, superintendents, patients, and themselves.[25] They were also to be upright and have an unblemished reputation. These ideals for nurses were adopted and naturalized by nursing students themselves. In 1920, nursing students at Severance Hospital organized a protest against the acceptance of a student with a background in the entertaining or *kisaeng* trade.[26] Female "chastity" was the most important virtue of women, they charged, and having a former *kisaeng* as a student, would disgrace the nursing profession.

In Japan, too, the education and profession of nursing from its inception was associated with and restricted to women. Missionary practices in nursing helped shape the profession, as the first formal nurse training institute in Japan was established in 1886 at Doshisha Hospital through the efforts of Protestant medical missionaries and Linda Richards, who is heralded as the United States' first professional nurse.[27] Nursing remained solidly a female vocation even as Japan's nursing field forged its own path tying nursing with war and imperialist expansion through the Red Cross and the experiences of nurses during the Russo-Japanese War. Government officials seized the opportunity to use the image of the nurse to advance ideals of patriotism and sacrifice. In the RG-period Grade 4 ethics textbook's Lesson 12, "The Red Cross," Florence Nightingale is presented as the epitome of benevolent charity and humanity, working tirelessly to comfort and assist the injured on the battlefield even at the risk of her own life, in turn respecting her patients for risking their lives for their nation, regardless of the side on which they fought.[28] This lesson is repeated throughout the colonial period in the GGK-published elementary school ethics textbooks in the lesson re-titled "Philanthropy" that identified nursing in its philanthropic beauty as an act of service to the nation.[29] This depiction, needless to say, masked the realities of the strict hierarchies in hospital work felt keenly by nurses charged with tasks from the very menial and tedious to laborious and exhausting.

Over time, Japanese terms and nursing practices took root in Korea as Japanese institutions came to dominate the training and employment of nurses in Korea. The RG consolidated hospital services, administration of public health measures (such as smallpox vaccination), and medical education at the Taehan Hospital, which trained and employed nurses called *kanhobu* with the female *pu* character that was in use in the Red Cross Hospital. The GGK solidified *kanhobu* as the official term for nurse with its Regulation for Nurses in 1914, which legislated nursing a female profession, thus eliminating the term *kanhowŏn* that missionaries had used.[30] The Regulation for Nurses stipulated not only that the holder of a nursing license be female but also that she be at least eighteen years of age, thereby limiting professional practice to only adult women.[31] A woman qualified for a nursing license if she either passed the GGK's nursing licensing exam or an exam administered at the provincial, county, or district level, or graduated from the nursing training program at the GGK Hospital, its charity-provincial hospitals, other public hospitals, the Japanese Red Cross Hospital, or another nursing training school approved by the GGK.[32] She was to possess no criminal record and be sound in mind and body. Moreover, similar to the requirements and conditions of nursing training programs in Japan, a nurse could lose her license if she was no longer sound in mind and body or displayed behavior that raised questions about her "good reputation." Nurses were to exemplify the "womanly virtues" as part of the Wise Mother, Good Wife ideal of womanhood incorporated in female education. Nursing students at training programs of public hospitals in colonial Korea were to possess "genuine humanity" with "gentle womanly behavior" and an "outward decorum of propriety and courtesy."[33] They learned housekeeping tasks of cooking, sewing, and laundering, skills they were to apply when caring for patients. Patients at public hospitals in colonial Korea held "feminine" expectations of nurses: they were to be unmarried and young. Rumors circulated that patients chose hospitals according to the attractiveness of their nurses.

The elevation of the profession of nursing did not happen overnight, of course. The marginal status of the missionaries' early nurse trainees ("ignorant, illiterate, deserted wives and widows who were usually homeless"[34]) was due in part to contact with men and negative associations of nursing with menial labor, for, according to one missionary, there was a "Korean notion that labor of any kind is low."[35] Moreover, many Korean women at the time were not literate or had received little education that would prepare them for a life preparing medications or studying physiology. The work was laborious and the training was rigorous and confining. Nursing students resided in the hospital or nursing school dormitory with twelve-hour-long work shifts in addition to their classroom learning, with little free time.[36] Indeed, they were to remain on the hospital grounds nearly full time, thus basically eliminating the possibility that women with domestic duties could receive proper training. The required conversion to Christianity at mission nursing schools or the use of Japanese language in training programs at public hospitals no doubt also limited the number of potential students.[37]

A Korean nurse's life was not easy. The nature of her work was so physically exhausting that nurses worked for only a few years until marriage, when their domestic duties would render their long shifts and dorm residence unfeasible. Some nursing students had difficulty adjusting to the lifestyle demanded by the regulations and routines of hospitals, which were different from other institutions with which they were familiar. The work also was mentally exhausting. At the lower end of the medical hierarchy, nurses had to respond to orders from attending physicians or their nursing superiors, though what they particularly resented was discriminatory treatment.[38] Larger hospitals, the sites of the most nursing education and employment opportunities, were the public facilities of the GGK and staffed overwhelmingly with Japanese personnel with whom Korean nurses sometimes clashed. Moreover, a Korean nurse's salary was a pittance, serving as no more than a supplement to her family's income.

Han Singwang, for example, described her years of nursing education as exceptionally grueling and discouraging. "I found no joy when I first began, wearing my white apron and cap over the blue nurse uniform, finding all the various tasks assigned by physicians such as [preparing and administering] medication bothersome."[39] Every four to five months, Han recalled, she would have night shift for a month, struggling to stay awake while sitting alone in a dark office, keeping her ears open for the sound of a ring from her patients. And she was fearful that patients would die, attending them so fervently that "sweat would fall even in the cold of winter." Of her experience when she had to handle and clean the corpses of patients who did not survive, "I cannot speak the fear." Missionaries' repeated assertions about the sacrosanct nature of nursing may well have been meant to encourage those who found aspects of the work distasteful.

Despite its drawbacks, nursing steadily attracted more recruits. For one, it was more readily available than other forms of higher learning such as teacher training and medicine.[40] Nursing and midwifery programs could be found throughout the country, such as at the public GGK Hospital, charity-provincial hospitals, mission hospitals in the two largest cities Seoul and Pyongyang, the Japanese Red Cross Hospital, and local private institutions. In the early years, a few charity hospitals offered a crash midwifery training course but these were phased out as nursing and midwifery training programs became standardized by the 1920s. In 1916, nursing and midwifery training programs were systematized in the major public hospitals in accord with the GGK Ordinance "Rules for Nursing and Midwifery Training at the GGK Hospital and Charity Hospitals," requiring only completion of common schools (four years' elementary education) for nursing applicants and graduation from a nursing program for midwifery, effectively tying midwifery to nursing education. Standards were raised after the educational reforms of 1922 to six years of common elementary and two years of higher common girls' school.[41] Upon completing their coursework, students would receive their respective licenses to practice.[42] The graduates did not need to pass an examination to qualify for their license. The nursing and midwifery training institute at the GGK Hospital was considered the most prestigious and attracted the majority of students.[43]

Even with the quotas on Korean students (capped at one-third of students) indicating that the main targets of nursing and midwifery training at public hospitals were Japanese women in the settler population, interested Korean students found nursing programs more accessible than medical education.[44] Nursing and midwifery training, in addition, did not require as many years as medical school—eighteen months for nurses, two years for midwives. Provided they met the educational and Japanese-language prerequisites, Korean women seeking a nursing or midwifery education did not need to study abroad. The emphasis on the practical curriculum in nursing schools allowed students to pay their own way. In lieu of tuition and fees, nursing students were to provide two years of hospital service upon graduation, thereby allowing those with fewer financial resources to receive higher education. Nursing students at mission training programs similarly could earn their educations. Both Han Singwang and Chŏng Chongmyŏng, who had families to support, recalled they chose nursing in part for that reason.[45]

THE NEW NURSE-MIDWIFE

In the West, childbirth's move away from the home to the hospital, overseen increasingly by male midwives and obstetricians, was a gradual one, catalyzed in part by developments in surgical techniques and antisepsis of the late nineteenth century. In Japan, reforms were undertaken to replace older childbirth practices seen as defiling and primitive in order to meet imperialist demands to increase the population with healthier bodies for industrial and military goals. Among these reforms was the standardization and professionalization of the New Midwife (*shinsanba*) that provided a gateway through which the state could supervise and intervene in Japanese women's reproductive activities.[46] In particular, the New Midwife was to oversee pregnancy to ensure safe delivery and recovery, as well as to prevent unregulated abortion and infanticide. Because midwifery was regarded as a specialization of nursing in Korea, with institutionally linked education, missionaries sometimes used the term nurse-midwife to refer to this new professional status.

In contrast to Japan and the West, Korea did not have much of a midwifery tradition before the twentieth century. Women gave birth at home, often with the assistance of a woman experienced in childbirth, a relative, friend, or neighbor.[47] Except for the *ŭinyŏ* appointed to the palace, women were not formally trained as midwives or to assist in childbirth. Being a birth attendant was not an occupation to which women devoted much of their time, or from which they derived their main source of income. Foreign missionaries in the late nineteenth century noted that these birth attendants tended to be widows, for customs discouraged elite or married women from interacting with men outside of their families.[48]

Settlers among the Japanese community in Korea, however, accustomed to having a midwife oversee deliveries increased the demand for trained (and primarily Japanese) midwives. This accounts in part for why the professional nurse-midwife in Korea was defined in the 1914 Regulation for Midwives as female by limiting holders of the midwife license to women. Except for cases that required surgical intervention, birthing remained in the female sphere.[49] Licensed midwives who received permission to practice had to have graduated from an accredited institution or successfully passed the midwifery licensing exam. Like nurses, they were bound to the same standards of physical fitness and moral character.[50] Regulations restricted midwives to "normal" pregnancies, and they were expected to seek a diagnosis from a physician if they suspected complications with the pregnancy or potential harm to the mother or fetus. When they came across a difficult delivery, they were to defer to physicians. Regulations also required midwives to report each delivery they oversaw, linking them to local administrative statistical projects on population growth and infant mortality. They, along with *ŭisaeng* and physicians, were granted the authority to write death certificates, including for stillbirths. Like physicians, midwives had to report to local authorities when opening or moving their practices. The fees they charged when they visited patients in their homes were set by the state.[51]

If a nursing student was fortunate and could obtain the means and time to receive additional schooling, she could prepare for a midwifery license, which promised to provide better opportunities. To qualify for the midwifery training program, candidates with a nursing degree had to demonstrate proficiency in Japanese language, mathematics, anatomy

TABLE 2.   Numbers of Licensed Nurses

	1910	1915	1920	1925	1930	1935	1940
Korean	17	21	47	101	182	419	780
Japanese	220	184	462	599	919	1,344	1,311
Foreign	3	10	10	21	19	20	7
Total	240	215	519	721	1,120	1,783	2,098

Source: *Chōsen sōtokofu tōkei nenpō* (various years).

TABLE 3.   Numbers of Licensed Midwives

	1910	1915	1920	1925	1930	1935	1940
Korean	20	5	21	66	173	424	649
Japanese	172	512	585	796	1,077	1,445	1,407
Foreign	0	0	0	0	1	0	1
Total	192	517	606	862	1,251	1,869	2,057

Source: *Chōsen sōtokofu tōkei nenpō* (various years).

and physiology, and nursing methods. An accelerated midwifery program was available to those who wanted to reduce their course time. But few institutions of higher learning beyond the higher common level were available for women in Korea, as discussed in earlier chapters, and many Japanese students in the settler population took the opportunity to study nursing in Korea rather than in Japan. This helps account for the fact that Japanese nurses continued to outnumber Korean nurses throughout the colonial period.

While the Japanese and GGK orientation of the nursing-midwifery training programs at the GGK Hospital or other public hospitals may not have appealed to Korean students, they nonetheless benefited from the exemption from the licensing exam that came with graduation. One of the founders of the Korean Nurses' Society, Chŏng Chongmyŏng, for example, decided to study midwifery at the GGK Hospital for this reason, even though she had graduated from the nursing program at Severance Hospital. When she graduated from the midwifery program in 1923, Chŏng was only one of three Korean women to receive a midwifery license.[52] But midwifery quickly became an attractive career choice for women, even more so than nursing and medicine. While the numbers of Korean nurses may have exceeded that of Korean midwives initially, the ratio between nurses and midwives became more balanced in the 1930s.[53]

Midwives had a nursing degree, but unlike nurses who worked long shifts in hospitals, midwives could open their own practices, work out of their homes, and have flexible hours.[54] It was possible for a woman to work while being married, having children, and maintaining a household. Han Singwang, for example, opened her own midwifery clinic in Masan after she married and had children.[55] Chŏng Chongmyŏng chose midwifery in order to support herself and her young son after being widowed.[56] Pak Chahye, the wife of renowned (and imprisoned and prematurely deceased) activist Sin Ch'aeho ran a clinic while raising her two young children alone.[57] Another former midwife recalled charging one *kama* of rice per delivery, which she likened to eight cows in present-day (2008) Korea.[58] Her first salary at a maternity hospital in Japan was forty-five yen, ten yen more than her grandfather, a college graduate, earned.[59] A female physician who had her own practice could have flexible hours, but maintaining a hospital or clinic, as discussed in an earlier chapter, was more demanding in terms of finances and equipment than a private midwifery practice. A midwife could just register with the local police station and put up a sign, her midwifery bag being the only equipment required. As with nursing, midwifery training was relatively accessible and of shorter duration, in contrast to physician training, making it more appealing to female students.[60]

This is not to say that the occupation was not filled with its own frustrations and difficulties. Some reported they felt underappreciated given their education and efforts.[61] Midwife Pak Chahye, for example, found difficulty attracting patients, sometimes going months without a patient.[62] While their practices may have offered flexibility, exhaustion came with the work as midwives received calls at unpredictable hours, sometimes late at night, with difficult labors that might last hours if not days. As one midwife recalled, although the Regulation for Midwives stipulated that they handle only "normal" cases, the reality was that women would often deliver on their own, calling in a physician only when complications arose.[63] Their clients' relative unfamiliarity with or reluctance to follow directives on what was deemed hygienic and proper natal care, and the stress produced by medically grave cases, could lead to disastrous consequences. For example, the *Tonga ilbo* reported in 1923 that neighbors physically assaulted midwife Ch'oe Hyosin and physician Chu Ryŏngsin, who Ch'oe had called in after the delivery faced complications, accusing them of causing the death of both mother and child after what appeared to be a successful delivery.[64] The neighbors blamed the deaths on the procedures of artificial resuscitation used during delivery.

The goal of colonial authorities was for a modern midwifery trained in biomedical obstetrics, with licensing and practices standardized and regulated by the state, in order to improve childbearing practices so as to mitigate maternal and infant mortality. Yet, as in the fields of medicine and nursing, structural barriers in public programs rendered midwifery training less accessible to Koreans, resulting in disproportionate numbers of Japanese midwives. For example, all instruction, exams, and hospital work were to be conducted in the Japanese language. The five-month midwifery crash course started in charity hospitals in the 1910s, while accepting Korean students, actively recruited students from among Japanese daughters of local military and regular police.[65] This not only ensured a source of Japanese midwives to serve the Japanese resident population, but also that whole families were involved in local public medical-health duties. GGK statistics indicate that throughout the colonial period, Japanese outnumbered Korean midwives.

Local (non-missionary, non-Japanese) efforts to establish a private educational institution to train Korean midwives in the months before Korea became a colony of Japan in 1910 included the "Midwife Training Institute" (Chosanbu yangsŏngso), which started with seventeen students, only to be closed a few months later due to funding issues.[66] The school resumed classes and graduated its first class of seven in 1913. It also offered lectures to the public and gained fame for delivering the daughter of the former king Kojong in 1912.[67] Unfortunately, financial constraints plagued the school and it finally closed for good in 1918. Moreover, not being an accredited institute meant its graduates could not receive a license to practice without passing a licensing examination. The GGK set strict accreditation standards for training schools.[68] Thus, even many mission medical training programs failed to receive accreditation. Severance was the first of the mission hospitals to gain accreditation for its nursing and midwifery programs but not until 1924. Even East Gate Women's Hospital did not have an accredited midwifery program, although it did offer midwifery courses for senior nurses.[69] Pyongyang Union Hospital received accreditation for its nursing-midwifery school in 1931.

COMPETING VISIONS

Missionary activities in nursing and midwifery evolved in the face of the challenge to their relevance posed by shrinking opportunities.[70]

Mission reports voiced frustration with the increasing oversight that impeded their medical work. Only Severance, among the mission hospitals, achieved accreditation as a medical school, but it first had to meet GGK demands, including higher credential requirements for professors. Licensing regulations steered potential medical and nursing missionaries away from Korea to China. One report attested to anxieties among missionaries over police interference and the new medical ordinances, which "hold[s] the power of life or death over the hospital."[71] The 1919 Private Hospital Regulation that required hospitals to have a separate isolation ward with at least ten beds was difficult to meet, so many mission hospitals shut their doors.

Furthermore, the options offered by the GGK and charity-provincial hospitals meant the loss not only of patients but also of personnel. Dr. Roy Smith of the Northern Presbyterian mission reported in 1917 that Japanese hospitals had more medical personnel on staff (in contrast to usually one at mission facilities), were able to treat three to five times more patients, and appealed to Koreans in that they were operated by Asians for Asians in "semi-Asian-style."[72] Missionaries competed not only with public hospitals that could handle many charity cases but also had private Japanese and Korean physicians.[73] Korean physicians and nurses left work at mission hospitals for better pay elsewhere.[74] The competition that medical missions faced from the changing colonial situation became so intense that in 1913 the Korean Medical Missionary Association admitted: "The establishment of medical work in many places in Korea by the Japanese government has caused some to think that this might seriously affect our medical missionary institutions, even perhaps to the extent of rendering the continuance of our work unadvisable, or at least to the point of making it unwise to plan any further enlargement of the present staff and equipment."[75]

By the 1920s, Mission Boards were displaying reluctance to support further medical work. This did not, however, lead missionaries to conclude that their work was no longer needed. Rather, they endeavored to strengthen medical mission facilities so as not to fall behind the standards and services of Japanese hospitals. "What if [Koreans] compare this apparent indifference to their needs with the diligence of the Japanese government in manning and equipping institutions for the sick?"[76] The Korean Medical Missionary Association in 1913 resolved that no new stations were to open unless they had at least two missionary physicians and a trained nurse with proper equipment. "Japanese medical work . . . greatly increases the urgency of a more efficient manning and equipment of our medical missionary plants."[77]

Moreover, there was a consensus among missionaries that they filled a spiritual void. Medical missions cultivated Christian workers who offered proper care, healing both the body and the soul in Christian service. In their view, while the government might be better at providing costly, "good, modern treatment and proper appliances," that did not relieve the church or mission boards of providing care for Korean patients. Dr. Weir exhorted, "No amount of Government Charity hospitals, no increase in the number of non-Christian doctors can in the least relieve the Church of Christ of her responsibility to the bodies as well as to the souls of men. . . . No, the work being done by the Government does not make ours less necessary, but more."[78]

Medical work for missionaries, thus, was foremost a moral mission. And, to stay relevant in a medical world dominated by the Japanese, they focused their attention on meeting the requirements set for them. This shaped the rationale for their services as well as the manner in which those services were provided. It also accounted in part for the condescension they exhibited toward Korean healing traditions, habits, and, occasionally, even the Koreans they trained. While missionaries strove to provide educational and professional opportunities to Korean women, their hospitals and nurse training programs were less than perfect in the eyes of their students and staff. Tensions between nurses and nursing students and administrators at mission hospitals or nursing training schools exploded on occasion in the form of nursing strikes.

In 1921, there was a general strike among Korean nurses at the Hall Memorial Union Hospital in Pyongyang in protest of harsh treatment and lack of proper social recognition from the missionary nurse supervisor.[79] Another nursing strike occurred in the same hospital a few years later in 1926.[80] In January 1924, a strike was organized at a hospital in Sunch'ŏn run by an American physician over the abysmally low income of nurses.[81] Two years later, in 1926, a Korean nursing student at East Gate Hospital training center committed suicide just shy of her graduation after being expelled for accidentally scalding a patient. The other nursing students were upset about the unilateral decision on the part of the American superintendent with little input or discussion from the students and demanded her removal. The previous year, the same superintendent apparently had expelled three other students.[82] This strike gained the sympathy of the Korean public, and the superintendent eventually had to leave. Nurses protested their working conditions at the GGK Hospital as well, exemplified by the nursing strike there in 1921.[83]

Yi Kkonme concludes that nursing strikes in general were class- and race-based conflicts protesting the inferior treatment nurses received as subordinates to their superiors. In the mission field, differences between Korean nurses and their missionary teachers and colleagues in vision or desire for the nursing occupation were perhaps best captured by the establishment of the two national professional nursing associations in the 1920s.[84] The KNA was formed in 1923 by missionary nurses associated with Severance Hospital. Its clear association with Christianity shaped the organization from the beginning. Annual meetings opened with hymns and Scripture readings and the Association voted that its membership committee should consist of foreign nurses (i.e., foreign missionaries) in charge of training schools. While its first purpose according to its constitution and by-laws was "to promote the spirit of mutual helpfulness among its members; to advance the interests of the nurse's calling," its second purpose was to spread "the gospel to the Korean people through the art of healing."[85] Korean nurses, so long as they were licensed, were welcome to join and to pay the same membership fee as required of foreign nurses.[86]

The KNA produced a publication, *The Bulletin of the Nurses' Association in Korea* (*Chosŏn kanhobu hoebo*; hereafter the *Bulletin*), in both English and Korean. The majority of the articles were written by missionaries with Korean translations, and, for the most part, the content of the two language sections overlapped. The *Bulletin* included minutes from its annual meetings, reports from various mission-run nurse training and public health programs, translations of articles from American nursing journals, medical cases, and various other public health education material.[87] KNA's major organizational activities centered on gaining official recognition as a branch of the International Council of Nurses (ICN). To accomplish this, the Association exhorted its members "to raise the standard of hospital training in Korea by the adoption of a uniform course of study." According to the *Bulletin*, the KNA submitted a request for membership at the ICN meeting in 1925.[88] Receiving the ICN evaluation that the KNA was "deficient as an Association," the KNA resubmitted its request in 1929, sending missionary Elisabeth Shepping and Korean nurses Yi Hyogyŏng and Yi Kŭmjŏn to represent KNA at the ICN meeting.[89] This time KNA was informed that it was denied membership because Korea was a colony of Japan and the ICN could not recognize both the Korean and Japanese branches. The ICN recommended that KNA join the Japanese Nurses' Association. In 1932, the KNA changed its name to match the name of the Japanese association and, together, they formed the Nurses' Association of the Japanese Empire, which gained ICN membership in 1933.[90]

What this suggests is that missionary nurses who formed the leadership of the KNA directed much of their focus toward meeting standards set for them by the GGK and ICN in the hope that gaining recognition would expand their activities and professional opportunities in a medical world that was slowly closing off to them. Translating a new series of textbooks, raising admission requirements (in 1926, the KNA voted to adopt the same standards as the GGK and provincial hospitals), and ensuring strict adherence to regulations in their nursing training programs, while all for the express purpose of improving the quality of nursing nonetheless centered on the tasks and needs of missionary nursing administrators. At best, this focus marginalized the concerns of individual nurses. At worst, it infringed on what Korean nursing students felt was acceptably fair.

Moreover, mission reports and the *Bulletin* betray the sense that, to missionaries, Korean nurses, while admirable, were not considered to be on the same par as foreign nurses. Although nominally the same in content, the Korean- and English-language sections of the *Bulletin* differed enough to suggest that although the organization was about "mutual helpfulness" with equal membership (as reflected by equal membership fees) it remained more didactic, with greater stress on the virtues and character of nurses, as well as medical educational material, in the Korean than in the English section. The December 1926 issue published an article only in the Korean section of the *Bulletin* that, while at first glance was a call for women's work and expanded freedoms, was also a reminder of the missionary vision of a womanhood of Christian modesty and service.[91] The same issue had the obituary of a Korean nurse who passed away while engaged in midwifery coursework that was not included in the English section, surprising if the association intended to foster a sense of community among its members.[92] An article explaining that God's salvation is attained through a spirit of service and sacrifice of self, again, did not appear in the English section.[93]

Whether the Korean section of the *Bulletin* was designed by missionaries or the Korean nurses who contributed to it is not clear. It is also possible that there was no time or personnel to translate articles written by Korean authors into English, hence their location in only the Korean sections of the *Bulletin*. Nevertheless, their content mirrored differences in the two member groups of KNA (Korean and missionaries) in general. Although by the mid-1920s nursing education in Korea was two decades old, none of the head nurses at mission hospitals were Korean.[94] In a chart of mission hospitals and dispensaries with their attached physicians and nurses, the names of Korean physicians and nurses are blatantly absent, although by then Koreans were heavily involved in mission medical work.[95] Missionaries were presented as instructors and administrators, while Korean nurses remained assistants and students. For example, the 1927 summer issue had a detailed report on the public health institute in Kongju in the English section of the *Bulletin* whereas the Korean version reprinted instructions on the proper feeding and care of infants, indicating that Korean nurses needed these instructions whereas foreign missionaries did not as they were connected to administrative work.[96]

Furthermore, the overall content of the *Bulletin* demonstrates its close connections to missionary-run institutions and programs and was relatively silent about events and issues in Korean society in general. The establishment of the Nurses' Society as a separate and Korean-run nursing organization suggests certain desires were not met by the KNA or mission medical institutions. KNA's reach and communication with the Korean populace were limited as it was a primarily foreign missionary–based organization. The founders of the Korean Nurses' Society, on the other hand, sought a Korean nursing organization that would be more active or at least a supplemental force in working with Koreans, particularly in rural areas. Unlike the missionary-led KNA, the Society was inclusive. There were no restrictions on membership besides having some form of nursing employment in a hospital, which would include nursing students as well as graduates who did not have a nursing license. All who qualified, whether in urban or rural areas, were encouraged to join.

Nursing was their "heavenly task" (*ch'ŏnjik*), Han Singwang stated at the Society's inaugural meeting. Not too dissimilar to missionary visions for nursing, Han urged members of the Society to follow the model of Florence Nightingale. However, the Society differed in that its goal was to enable the members' social (i.e., political) activity as nurses. It directed its focus toward the health education of families, care for orphans and the children of working women, and employment counseling services for nurses.[97] These activities point to the immediate interests of nursing students and recent graduates (i.e., jobs) and the platform of women's organizations of the time—cultural nationalist activities in education and leftist concern for the plight of the working class. To accomplish its goals, the Nurses' Society organized a health event open to the public in the summer of 1925, with musical entertainment (orchestra and vocal solos) and lectures given by physicians on swimming, the relationship between the body and mind, and venereal disease.[98] That same year, the Society also joined a flood disaster relief effort with two leftist women's organizations.[99] Unfortunately for the organization, there are no records of activity after 1925, indicating its demise. This may be due to the fact that Han Singwang, the chair of the Society, married in 1925 and left for Japan with her husband. Or perhaps the Society's leftist leanings or lack of funds made work difficult, a fate shared by other organizations of the time.[100]

"A BETTER BABY" MOVEMENT

Regardless of their differences, the Korean nurse-run Nurses' Society, the missionary-led KNA, and the colonial state shared an expressed commitment to the health education of families through women as mothers and housewives. Instructions in nursing and child-rearing through the domestic sciences curriculum at girls' higher common schools and print media, and the cultivation of women medical workers as physicians, nurses, and midwives were premised on the prescribed roles of women in the care and protection of their own health and that of their family members, particularly young children. This agenda is well exemplified by the case of infant health and social welfare projects.

By the 1920s, infant mortality statistics worldwide had become sensitive indices of social welfare and sanitary administration, resulting in a growing anxiety and the recognition that such rates needed to be lowered.[101] Yet despite the professed concern of the colonial authorities for the health and welfare of their ruled population, infant welfare work in Korea was woefully lacking. The state may have sought to enhance Korean women's reproductive health, which in turn was to strengthen the conjugal unit on which the imperial state was based, with its corollary of healthy infants and young children. But, as discussed earlier, midwives in colonial Korea were overwhelmingly Japanese and located in urban areas, largely serving the Japanese settler population. Korean women, moreover, continued in their reluctance to be examined by male physicians even though there was a dearth of female physicians.

Lack of funds and administrative burdens may account for the GGK's general negligence of maternal and infant welfare. However, comparisons with Japan and the shift toward increasing attention to maternal services after 1937 highlight characteristics of the medical system implemented in Korea in the 1920s and early 1930s. There were a number of educational facilities geared toward the training of female physicians in Japan, whereas none were implemented by the GGK in Korea. Midwives in Japan formed professional organizations, and local governments and private organizations instituted maternal health centers such as family planning and maternal clinics. Post-1937 policies to improve obstetric conditions and encourage reproduction in Korea included increasing food rations for pregnant women and day nurseries.[102] In general, limited health campaigns in Korea reflected an official attitude that medical services were foremost to serve imperial goals of conciliation, protect the Japanese settler community, and "offer" nominal health education, while access to medical care remained pitiably inadequate, especially in the countryside and for women and children.

It was in this vacuum that infant welfare centers in Korea were started, funded, and staffed overwhelmingly by foreign missionaries. Even before 1924, missionaries expended considerable effort on spreading their "gospel of hygiene"—especially as it related to everyday practices within the domestic space—whether from the pulpit, in hospitals and schools, through women's groups, printed literature, or other informal means. Tracts such as the "Care of Infants" written by Dr. James Van Buskirk were handed to mothers of small children in dispensaries. "Hygiene of Parturition" by Dr. Alfred M. Sharrocks and "Advice to Mothers" by Mattie Noble were used as basic texts in women's meetings and classes.[103] The women's mission hospital at East Gate was committed to teaching young mothers how to care for themselves and their babies and held infant welfare workshops with free baths and care during the summer months.[104]

Modeled on similar events in the United States, missionaries held baby shows—one record indicates as early as 1916 at the Songdo (Kaesong) Station—which offered awards to babies according to their sex, weight, height, proper number of teeth, and chest measurement. Missionaries used the shows to distribute educational information on the feeding, sleep, hygiene, and care of infants in the hopes to establish a "full fledged Better Baby Movement here and thereby help lessen the frightful mortality among infants."[105] In 1919, missionary Mabel Genso conducted a Mother's Club in Seoul to partake in this "Better Baby Movement," with monthly weighing and examination of infants and lectures by physicians and nurses.[106]

The work, however, was sporadic, dependent on interested missionary involvement, until it became systematic with the new infant health clinic at T'aehwa in 1924. T'aehwa pioneered a strong commitment to comprehensive social services by combining preventative and therapeutic medical care with an educational component, reinforced by home visits and return trips to the clinic. Babies attended periodically to be weighed, measured, examined, and treated for minor ailments. A Korean Bible woman or nurse, if available, provided a follow-up home visit. T'aehwa began a Baby Show in 1925, which became an annual event, spreading to other mission stations and was later conducted in conjunction with GGK-sponsored Children's Day. Missionaries offered free medical examinations, toys, and prizes for the "best" baby according to standards of weight, height, and health."[107]

Programs to assist pregnant women, infants, and children steadily expanded. Outpatient clinics opened in three different parts of Seoul.[108] Prenatal care was offered in conjunction with mission hospitals. Mothers registered with T'aehwa went to East Gate Women's Hospital for delivery, and Severance Hospital treated sick babies. Baths at T'aehwa started in 1927 for a nominal fee, and then water was let loose for street children in exchange for recitation of Bible verses.[109] A year later, in 1928, T'aehwa began a milk-feeding station that prepared and provided undernourished infants with supplementary nutrition. As it was soon discovered that some mothers found the notion of their children drinking milk from an animal abhorrent, a soy milk formula from China was used. The soy milk formula was deemed successful for catering to the dietary tastes of Koreans and, being more affordable to produce, T'aehwa even secured a government permit to can soy milk powder.[110]

Women's and infant health care thus came to the forefront of cooperative medical mission ventures in the late 1920s. T'aehwa hosted the first public health conference in 1926, inviting nurses and midwives across denominations and from around the peninsula to come for lectures on hygiene and public health work with mothers and children. This became an annual event called the Public Health Nurses' Institute that was held at various infant welfare centers throughout the peninsula. In 1928, the Korean Women's Medical Training Institute opened its doors and devoted itself to the medical education of Korean women. The following year, T'aehwa joined forces with Severance Hospital and East Gate Women's Hospital to create the Seoul Child-Welfare Union with Dr. Douglas Avison, a pediatrician at Severance, as its director. The three sites shared personnel and resources, with a Well-Baby Clinic at each. The clinics also served to train nursing and medical students in public health work. This was the same year that Ewha inaugurated its Home Economics Department. According to one of its faculty, a Korean graduate of mission schools, Home Economics was directly linked with efforts to reduce infant mortality and thus the same instruction on infant care given to mothers attending infant welfare clinics was given to Home Economics students.[111] Furthermore, a printed list of publications endorsed by the KNA for the edification of Korean nurses included health tracts given to mothers at the infant welfare clinic.[112]

Other mission stations throughout the country followed suit with similar programs. Missionary Maren Bording started the infant and maternal health clinic in Kongju in 1924, and opened a new branch in Taejŏn when the provincial capital moved there from Kongju in 1932. Medical work at the Kongju clinic differed from other mission stations in that it lacked a doctor and hospital but housed a full-service infant and maternal health center. Besides a bimonthly Well-Baby Clinic, Kongju started a Milk Station in 1927 and a nursery for motherless babies or babies of sick mothers in 1930. It also offered a two-year training course for infant-care nurses targeting high school girls and a four-month post-graduate nursing course in Public Health and Infant Welfare. There was a clinic for Japanese babies, and a Korean nurse-midwife was on staff devoted to the prenatal, delivery, and postnatal care of Korean mothers and babies in their homes.[113]

While acknowledging the inferior state of public works and family finances, missionaries attributed early childhood mortality largely to maternal ignorance—particularly with regard to feeding—fueled by Korean customs. Mothers, in their view, did not know the proper methods of feeding and failed to offer nutrition required for healthy growth. Late weaning and the lack of milk after weaning, the inferior quality of the Korean diet (as missionaries perceived it), pre-mastication of food (transferred from adults' mouths to infants), the early introduction of solid food (while still breastfeeding), restrictions in diets of sick children, and feeding infants on demand instead of on schedule, were said to tax the health of infants through their digestive tracts, exacerbating or even bringing on illnesses that could lead to an untimely demise. Missionaries thus focused on proper nutrition and eating habits, particularly the scheduled feeding of infants, as the root of most infant illnesses. The Kongju Infant Welfare Center handed out a feeding schedule pamphlet written in vernacular Korean to mothers. The rhetoric of the pamphlet was frightening: "44 out of 100 newborns are dead in their first two years," it warned. The reasons lay in the inability to adhere to scheduled feeding, clean bathing, and clean clothing. "Do you want to kill your beloved child?" the pamphlet asked, "Or do you want it to live?"

While infant welfare work in Europe and America retreated from a focus on milk supply to focus instead on labor legislation (to enhance breastfeeding), free meals to supplement breastfeeding mothers' nutrition, and mothers' pensions, missionaries in Korea continued to concentrate their efforts on changing Korean child-rearing customs, particularly in terms of diet. They circulated detailed instructions on solid foods in addition to scheduled feeding. Korean children were "fortunate" if they survived habits that allowed them to "eat nearly all kinds of green fruit and vegetables," only to suffer from the intestinal parasites contracted from the not-so-dead-and-dried-fish at the markets.[114] Perhaps because breastfeeding was nearly universal, missionaries felt little need to mention its benefits, although they were disquieted by the fact that Korean infants seemed to nurse constantly for three to four years, well beyond the recommended one year. Missionaries may have invoked poverty, poor sanitation, and improper pre- and postnatal care as matters of concern, but they did not pursue these aspects of infant welfare work with as much fervor as they did Korean feeding habits.

By the late 1930s, mission infant welfare work existed in some shape or form in Seoul, Taejŏn, Kongju, Andong, Kangye, Taegu, Sinch'ŏn, Pyongyang, Haeju, Chemulp'o, Wŏnsan, Kaesŏng, Chŏrwŏn, Ch'unch'ŏn, and Suwŏn. The expansion of this new field of medical work, however, seemed precarious in a time of retrenchment. For example, even when financial support was offered to expand or develop hospitals, as in the case of Ms. Schauffler who was considering in the mid-1920s whether to donate more funds to the Cornelius Baker Memorial Hospital in Andong named after her father, the Mission Board refused, not wanting to commit to sustaining hospitals at expanded levels.[115] They also expected medical missions to be self-supporting. By the 1920s, the North Methodists had closed three of their six medical stations. Medical missions in Pyongyang decided to consolidate their efforts through union work with one hospital.[116]

Medical work was heavily dependent on personnel and funds— should the physician or nurse go on furlough, mission hospitals closed unless they were able to procure replacements, often employing Korean graduates to serve in the interim. The global economic recession of the 1930s further reduced appropriations, and missionaries often had to dig into their own pockets or appeal to personal friends and supporters to fund their clinics. Well-Baby clinics required a doctor's time—precious when doctors at mission stations were already overtaxed.[117] Clinics demanded a full-time nurse when few could be spared, and someone, preferably Korean, to communicate with mothers. Space was an issue, with even church offices put to use if there was no room at the hospital or dispensary. Milk was not inexpensive either; the center at Kongju had to turn to serving a more upper-class clientele in order to fund its milk service, thereby deviating from the professed goal of social service for the poor.[118]

The efforts at times seemed to cost too much with too little result. The Well-Baby clinic in Andong shut down for a few years in the early 1930s for this reason. According to its annual report, "One of our saddest set-backs has been the dropping away of the baby clinic. It was found that we were giving too much charity."[119] Nevertheless, despite the strain on resources, by 1940 most Presbyterian and Methodist mission stations offered some form of infant welfare services.

CARVING A SPACE

Situating mission infant welfare work within the larger context of global missions and Korea's colonial medical system furthers our understanding of why health services for infants were promoted in a period of declining resources. Medical work, in general, was believed to be an essential part of Christian work, even "an outgrowth of Christianity."[120] In the mid-1920s, the Rockefeller Foundation sponsored the Laymen's Inquiry, which produced a report representing seven American Protestant denominations that assessed the work of and suggested reforms for Protestant missions. It reflected the unease Protestant denominations felt about the role of Christianity and missions, particularly in Asia, and the relationship between evangelism and social service. Moreover, it addressed concerns about whether medical missions were needed where imperial powers proactively constructed modern medical systems, as in the case of Japan in Korea. The report acknowledged, "With a Government so progressive, and so intent on making the best of western science its own, there has seemed to other boards little need of embarking upon a costly program of medical relief."[121] However, the report concluded that this did not signal the end of medical mission work. Rather, the report justified mission work as necessary to realize the ideal of Christian service in Korea.

This was founded on the conviction that Christianity in Korea offered different and better modes of medical service and education. While acknowledging GGK improvements in Korea's sanitary and medical administration, missionaries were critical of Japanese medicine, revealing tensions that blurred the line between cooperation and competition. Missionaries claimed to provide moral and spiritual dimensions to modern ways of being that Japan's colonial project of material and technological modernization lacked. One mission hospital reported, "As Government institutions and native physicians increase and as the church grows the purpose and need of the mission hospital changes from its importance as a means of contact more and more to that of the Good Samaritan."[122] Medical education at Severance was essential for it offered "medical education under Christian influence and in the Christian spirit." Imagine the danger then, as Dr. Van Buskirk, a professor at Severance continued, "if we fail to do this . . . we allow the great and influential medical profession to fall into non-Christian or anti-Christian hands."[123]

Missionaries feared that a "Japanese system of medical treatment, empirical remedies, shot-gun prescriptions, and intra-cutaneous, intramuscular, intra-venous, and intra-anything injections" would let the "lust for gold" rule the work of the physician.[124] In such a system, "it is only the charity patient who is being turned away." To counter this, Christian physicians and schools producing Christian medical workers instilled "the spirit of Christian Service" to bring about "the milk of human kindness." Thus, the future of medical missions was to lie in public health, particularly with social services as an extension of "the usefulness of the hospital by connecting its helpful service with the homes of the people."[125] Medical missions were to ensure Koreans' access to medical services that might be hampered by material, economic, or social conditions, through the provision of care in the home "as a practical expression of the gospel of Christ." The Laymen's Inquiry concurred: "the Commissioners are convinced that . . . much that is worthwhile can be done in [fields of health education, preventive medicine, and public health nursing]. . . . In particular, efforts in health education should be focused upon school children and mothers."[126]

For these reasons, medical missionaries insisted on the value of their presence. Keeping to their Christian mandate, they persevered to continue medical services by meeting GGK licensing and operating requirements, particularly in areas of common interest such as infant welfare. In this way, there was a tacit partnership between the missionaries and the colonial authorities. The 1927 mission Public Health Conference included a visit to the Government Hospital.[127] Mission-affiliated visiting nurses and midwives used the sort of Midwife Bag that was used in Japan.[128] It was said that "government officials approve highly of anything done for public health," and that the work in Kongju was "shown much consideration by them."[129] The milk station in particular was supported by the local police and higher officials.[130]

Infant welfare work in Kongju (and later Taejŏn) demonstrates most clearly this relationship between medical missions and the colonial state. Director Maren Bording was permitted a new building to house the infant welfare work by local authorities in 1929. To conduct her work, Bording was granted a medical license although she was not a trained physician.[131] The state also made annual contributions starting in 1930. As children of Japanese officials registered at her clinic, the local government loaned a small building for a milk station so that milk would not have to be transported daily from Kongju to Taejŏn. At other centers, Japanese support came as single donations, such as the fifty yen received from Countess Kadama, wife of the vice governor of Korea in 1932, to be used for prizes in the Baby Show in Seoul, or serums to vaccinate children. If tensions existed with the colonial government in the carrying out of infant welfare work, mission records are relatively silent on the subject.[132]

Missionaries saw infant welfare as a need not fully met by the state. While the GGK established an elaborate system of hospitals and medical education throughout the peninsula and proclaimed various public health campaigns, GGK campaigns, in fact, lacked the resources to effect significant material improvements in Korea's health conditions. The poor state of public works (such as open sewers) in Korea did not help matters, but until proper infrastructure could be implemented, missionaries sought public health work as a means to "preach prevention and prevent sickness."[133] The state, through its social service arm, the *Chōsen shakai jigyōkai* (Korean Welfare Society), began to sponsor a Children's Day in 1928, three years after T'aehwa began its annual Baby Show. This was later extended in 1931 to an annual weeklong public education campaign in May termed "Loving and Protecting the Child" (K. *yuyu-a aeho*; J. *nyūyoji aigo*). But while the activities of the Korean Welfare Society were generally limited to working with other medical institutions to provide free health and dental exams for the young and publicizing the proper health care of infants, standard weight and height charts, and statistics on infant mortality, missionaries endeavored to work directly with their Korean clients on a frequent, long-term basis. Despite the annual exhortations of the "Loving and Protecting the Child" campaigns, infant welfare institutions failed to materialize in a significant way in the 1930s. In 1936, there were around twenty infant welfare–related institutions and day-care centers, most of them run by Christian missionaries.[134]

What the growing emphasis on missionary infant welfare activities meant for Korean nurses and midwives was greater opportunities for professional development. To increase the number of midwives, for example, the East Gate Women's Hospital started a special training session for senior nurses in midwifery in 1929, equipping the classroom in the same way as the GGK Hospital training program for midwives and employing the same teacher in the hope that their graduates would pass the government licensing examination and become licensed midwives.[135] The expanding possibilities are illustrated by individual cases such as that of Han Singwang. It was Han's work at T'aehwa that enabled Elma Rosenberger to gain access to and be able to communicate with Korean mothers.

Another integral figure in infant welfare work was Frances Lee (Yi Kŭmjŏn) who replaced Han in assisting missionaries at T'aehwa. T'aehwa later financed Lee's study abroad in the graduate Public Health program at the University of Toronto in 1929.[136] She returned to Korea and was active in infant welfare work in Kongju with Maren Bording. Lee used her experience and position to produce educational material for Korean women not only for use in the clinic but also in Korean print media. It was she who wrote the informational materials in Korean to be passed out at the clinics. She also occasionally published on infant care in women's journals. In Kongju, Lee was the midwife who went on rounds to handle the prenatal care of Korean mothers, a novel practice at the time.

Mothers' Meetings were another central component of infant welfare work. While mission personnel may have been involved and sometimes called in to speak with mothers, the day-to-day business of these gatherings could not have been sustained without the leadership of Korean nurses such as Kim Tai Hyung at Kangkei.[137] The input and leadership of Korean women were also important to operating activities connected to the clinics. Mothers, themselves, took leadership roles in Cradle Roll (a roster in churches of infants visiting infant welfare centers) activities and in mothers' groups. Some became so well versed in medical procedures that they would demand that the attending physician examine their child with a stethoscope, even though, due to the large number of patients waiting to be seen, most physicians would have preferred to simply check the health status of a child based on height and weight charts.[138] It was the pressure from Korean mothers about their dietary preferences and the financial difficulties involved in traveling to infant welfare centers that prompted missionaries to develop their soy milk formula and to open outpatient clinics in other parts of the city.

Over time, Korean medical workers played an increasingly important role in child welfare activities. Korean women contributed articles on women's and children's health issues to the Christian newspaper, *Kidok sinbo*.[139] When mission personnel were stretched, on furlough, or simply not available, Korean physicians, such as Dr. Kim at East Gate, took over the responsibilities of conducting examinations at the clinics. Moreover, as infant welfare centers developed social service functions, such as the kindergarten at T'aehwa, they trained Koreans who were to play important roles in the post-1945 period: for example, Esther Koh (Ko Hwanggyŏng), whose education, experience, and activities in girls' education and the social welfare of mothers and children in the Inch'ŏn area of the late 1930s and 1940s helped garner her a position as the only female member of Park Chung Hee's advisory committee on family planning in the early 1960s.

For the most part, the GGK condoned missionary infant welfare activities. The missionaries' fragile partnership with the authorities in the realm of medicine, however, restricted their activities. Moreover, their belief in the shared goals of civilization tacitly tied them to imperial goals of conciliation and nominal health education, thereby re-inscribing gendered norms for women's participation in health professions and activities. Missionaries thus failed to muster a movement to sufficiently address the structural factors contributing to infant mortality, a concern many Korean reformers raised in the press. Moreover, they promoted Christian visions for womanhood, nursing, and medicine that may not have appealed to everyone. The missionaries' legacy is not best measured by the number of infants examined and treated, or the mothers who converted to the new regimes in child-rearing or even Christianity. Rather, what the missionaries bequeathed was a firm rationale for, model of, and experience in infant welfare work. The leadership experience gained by Korean women as medical and social service professionals and organizational leaders left an indelible mark as some women took up leadership positions in rebuilding Korean society after its liberation from Japanese colonial rule.[140]

CHAPTER 4

Negotiating Gynecology

Constant Imperatives, Evolving Options

In a 1909 report on women's medical work, Rosetta S. Hall commented that one of the more frequent conditions among her patients at the mission woman's hospital in Pyongyang was "women's disease."[1] "Women's diseases," she recorded, were not only time-consuming and difficult to treat, but distinct, demanding new forms of medical interventions. She continued, "although we have all varieties of gynecological work in Korea, and have had some most unique cases, that we believe our Professors of this subject at home never saw or heard of, the most common complaint of all that comes to us is for some form of childlessness. Because of the high death rate in infancy and early childhood, and the prevalence of Confucian ideas concerning the necessity of male progeny, many women are childless here who would not be considered so in the home-land." Hall's observations about her patients' medical concerns and the family customs that privileged male progeny highlight the link between what was termed "women's disease" or *puinbyŏng* (婦人病) and infertility. It also points to anxiety about infant mortality, conventionally associated with pediatrics and obstetrics, as corollaries of gynecology. News of patients' successful pregnancies after consulting Hall or other physicians like her drew increasing numbers of patients to the new hospitals.[2] By 1917, gynecological cases outnumbered all other cases at the mission women's hospital in Pyongyang.[3]

Several years later in 1924, the Seoul Youth Association sponsored a public debate on birth control. The daily newspaper *Tonga ilbo* duly observed that birth control as a topic to be discussed publicly was unprecedented in Korea.[4] A female commentator reflecting on this event a few months later recalled the joy she felt listening to the arguments. Although she was not able to attend the entire event, she sympathized with the position of those who promoted birth control as a means of liberating women from the unproductive labor of bearing many children.[5] Her voice was the start of many in a growing call for *sana chehan* or *chojŏl*—the limitation, management, or regulation of birth—that took shape in Korean print media in the 1920s and 1930s. Influential figures, predominantly men, from various sectors including education, religion, medicine, journalism, law, and social activism weighed in with their opinions. Women did as well, including those who sought to actively practice birth control in their daily lives.

While these two cases suggest opposing agendas—the former to promote women's fertility, the latter to curb it—they were both rooted in similar reproductive politics: the desire to affect outcomes in matters of pregnancy, childbirth, and child-rearing. Despite limitations in the availability of patient case histories and statistical documentation of *puinbyŏng*, abortion, and use of contraceptives or fertility techniques, examining what is said by and about women as well as their consumption of health-related services and products provides us with insights into women's health-related afflictions, treatment, and experiences. In particular, women's attempts to control their reproduction, while drawing from an arsenal of modern and traditional resources, converged with the pronatalist interests of the colonial state and Korean patriarchal family norms. The emphasis on women's reproductive health in gynecology re-inscribed women's care-providing roles in their capacities as mothers.

DEFINING *PUINBYŎNG*, UNDERSTANDING THE FEMALE BODY

The easing of restrictions on publications and assembly in the 1920s led to an expanding print culture in which emerged a growing discussion of the nebulous disease category *puinbyŏng*. These discussions were printed primarily in women's journals and columns in daily newspapers but also appeared in literature for general audiences. A study of the women's column in the *Chosŏn ilbo* from 1924 to 1950 found that 63.3

percent of the total 2,410 articles dealt with hygiene and medical care in the home, with 95 percent of those articles published between 1924 and 1935.[6] The column explained illnesses such as venereal diseases, tuberculosis, Hansen's disease, digestive ailments, and smallpox and other similar contagions. It advised special precautions to take in particular seasons (for example, summer as a time of dangerous digestive ailments; winter for coughs and colds). Basic individual health-promoting activities (breathe fresh air, drink boiled water, engage in moderate exercise), care for one's teeth, and child-rearing techniques were other common topics. What also emerged in these articles was a growing discussion of new sexual knowledge, particularly as it related to reproduction. Articles on sex education (including male and female reproductive systems), hormones, venereal diseases, infertility, pregnancy and childbearing techniques, postpartum care, birth control, and the female menstrual cycle frequently appeared in newspapers and journals, often written by physicians (both those trained in biomedicine and those in *hanbang*) and social reformers (particularly in making the case for or against birth control or sex education in schools).

The image presented in these articles is of the inherently pathological nature of women's bodies. Women were defined by their reproductive organs, particularly their wombs, the Korean term being literally "housing the child." These wombs, the site of menstruation and the conception, gestation, and delivery of infants, often produced strange discharges, pains, menstrual irregularity, and abnormal growths or protrusions that were generally placed under the rubric *puinbyŏng*.[7] Agreement on a precise definition of *puinbyŏng* proved difficult, as writers often differed in their training, backgrounds, and professional positions, but, in general, as gynecologist Hŏ Sin asserted, *puinbyŏng* referred to disorders that affected women's internal organs—the uterus, ovaries, Fallopian tubes, and peritoneum.[8] It thus often was conflated with the term *chagungbyŏng* or "uterine disease." Other gendered conditions such as hysteria, *hwabyŏng* ("fire illness," a nervous disorder understood in both psychiatry and *hanbang*), and childbearing were of concern insofar as they related to afflictions of a woman's reproductive organs.[9] More importantly, *puinbyŏng* not only specified a particular constellation of ailments limited to the female sex, but also indicated that the patients concerned were mainly married women in their childbearing years, or females who would become future wives and mothers.

This correlates with the gynecological tradition during the Chosŏn dynasty that aimed to treat married women in their reproductive years. Nuns and widows, children and the elderly, were not included in this category, and their diseases were thus addressed differently.[10] Called *pugwa* (Ch. *fuke*), Sino-classical gynecology and its correlative medical theories are better understood as "medicine for women" that details "a changing repertory of therapies" for disorders specific to "wives" (*pu* refers to a married woman), including those recommended for "birth" or what we today would consider to be obstetrics. A female's normality revolved around her reproductive capability, signified by her menstrual cycle, and treatment with medications was prioritized over other methods.[11] The early twentieth-century emphasis on afflictions of women's reproductive organs shifted the understanding of sexual difference, and the understanding of female normality became informed by an anatomical model of the body. What emerged in health-related articles in newspapers and journals in the early twentieth century was a female body defined most prominently by its reproductive organs (ovaries, uterus, Fallopian tubes) and function (reproduction). As gendered production and consumption of hygienic knowledge situated women as mothers responsible for the health of their children, they also were expected to care for their own bodies, central to which was the care of their reproductive health.

Puinbyŏng as a term or specific health concern appears in many titles of health-related articles targeting women in the early twentieth century. While physicians today reflecting on this period may associate *puinbyŏng* with inflammation of the female reproductive system stemming from disease or infection, discussions in the colonial period print media nearly always mentioned women's menstruation, continuing the centrality of the female reproductive processes from earlier traditions of gynecology.[12] Hŏ Sin maintained that *puinbyŏng* did not affect girls before menarche unless it was determined after its diagnosis in adulthood that the patient was afflicted with a congenital problem, injury, or underdevelopment of her reproductive organs before puberty.[13] Women, popular media urged, were to become aware of their monthly cycles and monitor their discharges, which were intimately related to their reproductive processes. Women were also told they were the weaker sex and had to take more precautions than men as they were more prone to afflictions and their ailments were more difficult to treat.[14] Failure to receive immediate diagnosis and treatment for any menstrual disorder or prolonged discharge, physicians warned, could lead to infertility and even death.

For women, an understanding of one's own menstruation became essential. Menses—assessed based on age at onset, duration, frequency, amount of flow, accompanying pains or other ailments, and regularity—was at the root of what was defined as "normal." Its mutual connection to other bodily processes meant that trouble elsewhere in the body could affect one's cycle and that menstrual disorders in turn could incite other ailments such as hysteria. Cessation or too little flow, whether it was heavy or dark, intense pains, foul odor, irregular cycles, absence before the age of eighteen—all warranted concern. Furthermore, as one's cycle was intimately connected with one's state of mind, mental or emotional disturbances or the delusion that one was pregnant (phantom pregnancy) could temporarily stop menses. It also was held that mental instability brought about by menstrual disorders could lead to female criminal behavior.

Menstrual disorders and uterine diseases had a central place in late nineteenth- and early twentieth-century medical texts and health manuals for women in the West, where an emphasis on women's menstruation was fundamental in the medical specialty of gynecology and in the etiology of women's ailments. Anatomical understanding of the body enabled the synecdoche of woman with her uterus, and gynecology dealt "with the pathologies of women's reproductive organs, or in the functional language of endocrinology as the science of regulating the female hormone system."[15] Physicians saw a woman "as the product and prisoner of her reproductive system," which determined her mental and physical capacities, duty in life (breeder of children), as well as her nervous system, believed to be intimately connected with the uterus.[16] Hence, the medical examination of a woman began and ended with her uterus, seen as the root cause of her physical and mental ailments.[17] According to a late nineteenth-century medical dictionary in the United States, the diseases of women were generally defined as "those morbid processes and mechanical deviations of which the principal seat is in the sexual system, that is, in the ovaries, uterus, and breasts," the majority of which ailments occurred in women's reproductive years.[18]

The Korean colonial discourse on *puinbyŏng* and menstruation shared similarities with its predecessors and contemporaries across the seas. Many writers trained or worked at mission hospitals, the GGK medical training institutes, or abroad and were familiar with the biomedical model of the body and the gynecological emphasis on the female reproductive organs. In fact, in Korea, menstruation was what defined womanhood. Particular to women, it was what made them different from men.[19] The monthly flow of blood indicated a woman's fertility, and thus her womanhood. Physicians went so far as to assert that women who did not bear children would experience menopause at a much younger age, even in their thirties, as their reproductive organs would fail to function if they did not fulfill their natural destiny as women. Menopause, the cessation of menstruation, did not simply signal an end to a woman's reproductive functions but the loss of womanhood and femininity altogether.[20] Postmenopausal women, it was said, became like men, and *puinbyŏng* did not affect them except in cases of physical injuries such as fistulas. Menopause, or afflictions not related specifically to women's reproductive function, received only cursory attention.[21]

Puinbyŏng, as it related to menstrual disorders, can be roughly divided as follows: absence (amenorrhea), irregularity, and excessive pain. Menarche (onset of menses) was one area of interest among medical researchers and, in fact, several surveys throughout the colonial period were conducted to determine and evaluate the age of onset of menstruation in Koreans.[22] In 1931, Yun Ch'iwang, a physician at Severance Union Medical College, published his research finding that menarche for the majority of Korean girls came between thirteen and sixteen years of age, although he saw a wide range from ten to twenty-four years of age. Physicians warned that menarche was an unstable time, particularly during the bodily and emotional transitions of puberty. Improper hygiene or failure to provide sex education for young girls, it was contended, invited a host of problems, whether it be the pelvic inflammations of *puinbyŏng*, nervous disturbances brought about by the shock or fear girls experience when they first menstruate, or even indecent sexual behavior as they began to experience desire for the other sex. Age at onset depended on environment, lifestyle, and constitution.[23] Warmer climates and urban lifestyles brought on earlier menarche, as did healthier constitutions. Late onset, however, was not much of a concern until eighteen, at which point its absence indicated underdevelopment or lack of function in reproductive organs or other serious ailments such as malnutrition, anemia, jaundice, drug addiction, tuberculosis or other contagious disease.[24]

Another concern women were to be on the lookout for was the sudden cessation of menstruation after menarche and establishment of a regular cycle, but without pregnancy or breastfeeding. This amenorrhea could result from (1) blockage at the cervix, (2) underdevelopment or injury to the uterus or ovaries, (3) extreme stress on the body, or (4) phantom pregnancy.[25] Cervical blockage would prevent the menstrual flow from draining, and the obstruction could result from injury (from a beating or childbearing) or childhood illness such as scarlet fever, smallpox, or diphtheria. Underdevelopment or injury to the uterus or ovaries stemmed from insufficient nutrition or poor health, and infections or growth (such as cysts or tumors), which would interfere with their functions. Malnutrition, overwork, fatigue, and a serious disease, such as tuberculosis, were other possible factors. Knowing the cause of one's amenorrhea would allow one to seek proper treatment. For example, the severe pain that often accompanied cervical blockage could be rectified by surgery.

Temporary amenorrhea, when menses were several days early or late or skipped months, signaled irregularity (*pulsun*). Irregularity was to be carefully monitored and treated, as it adversely affected women's fertility. Other irregularities or abnormalities expressed themselves in excessive pain, heavy menstruation, spotting between cycles, or long duration beyond seven days. Excessive pain was especially troublesome for it not only indicated some other affliction, but also could grate on one's nerves and patience, thus inviting hysteria. Physicians suggested that these symptoms signaled a multitude of troubles, from growth of cysts or tumors in the reproductive organs to a prolapsed uterus brought about by poor postpartum care that did not allow for stretched ligaments to recover properly, presence of some pelvic inflammation or infection, anemia, or plain exhaustion of the body.

Another major symptom of *puinbyŏng* and subject of much discussion was *taehajŭng* ("symptoms below the waistline"), which referred to the various nonmenstrual discharges that a woman might experience. Roughly translated as leukorrhea ("the whites"), a similar concept existed in American tocological thinking and was attributed to pelvic inflammations. The term *taeha* stems from the Sino-classical medical tradition. In earlier times, gynecologists were called *taeha ŭi*, as they mainly treated women for their secretions, and a practitioner's reputation depended on how well he was able to treat women for *taehajŭng*. In twentieth-century medical thinking, *taeha* signified a symptom and not a disease in and of itself, although women who had such trouble would be labeled as being afflicted with *puinbyŏng*.[26] A constant flow of secretions from the uterus, heavy enough to soak pads, and ranging in color from clear to white, yellow, and red, was deemed *taeha* and might or might not be accompanied by pain or fever. Even biomedical physicians used the term *taeha* or noted that their patients did. For them, *taeha* indicated inflammation in the pelvis, uterine membranes, ovaries, or Fallopian tubes. It could be a simple bacterial infection brought about by poor hygiene or contraction of a venereal disease such as gonorrhea or syphilis. In the worst case, *taeha* revealed cancer.

As this discussion suggests, a continuation of earlier terms and knowledge of women's bodies and ailments was interwoven within the modern field of gynecology as it was taking shape. How, for their part, did *ŭisaeng* practitioners during the colonial period understand and treat *puinbyŏng*? On the one hand, they inherited a scholarly medical tradition related to "medicine for women" that aimed to enhance and protect women's fertility. The *puin* (literally, "married woman") chapter of the *Tongŭi pogam*, a classical text in Chosŏn scholarly medicine, opens with, "The way of life begins with the birthing of children, and having children first requires that the menses be regular."[27] Managing one's secretions—both menstrual and *taeha*—was one of the chapter's major focuses.

On the other hand, *ŭisaeng* could not ignore biomedical knowledge on which they were examined in order to receive a *ŭisaeng* license to practice. While *ŭisaeng* on the whole rejected a biomedical universalism that excluded traditional medicine *in toto*, they held no unified opinion on a definitive standard or a curriculum of knowledge regarding medicine and the body. Their positions varied on whether a universal medicine should contain both Western and Eastern medicines, whether Eastern medicine should be understood as complementary to Western medicine, whether aspects of Eastern medicine had biomedical validity, or whether acupuncture and moxibustion could be likened to chiropractics or osteopathy. The *ŭisaeng* journals themselves reveal different interests and varied voices. Some published translations of biomedical treatises and invited physicians in the biomedical tradition to submit articles.[28] Pieces submitted by traditional practitioners ranged from expositions on Chinese traditional medicine, identification of areas where *hanbang* could complement or even be superior to biomedicine, calls to improve *hanbang* through the establishment of organizations (as mentioned in chapter two), educational facilities, and research agendas, reprints of the *ŭisaeng* regulations, and case studies.[29]

Gynecological information in *ŭisaeng* journals and study guides for the licensing exam presented *puinbyŏng* as a pathology of women's reproductive organs.[30] *Ŭisaeng* were to understand the etiology of endometrial infections, menstrual disorders, and sexually transmitted diseases, as well as the physiology of women's reproductive system and pregnancy. But traditional therapeutics and understanding of illness could also be part of a larger repertoire in the treatment of *puinbyŏng*. For example, *hanbang*-based prescriptions were listed among treatments for "morning sickness," an ailment highlighted in both biomedical and *hanbang* traditions.[31] In addition, moxibustion was claimed to result in the successful conception and delivery of a child even when the patient's infertility was determined to be attributed to biomedical understandings of inflammation or physical abnormalities such as a prolapsed uterus.[32] It is easy to see how an already established gynecological tradition that focused on menstrual regularity and fertility could segue into a biomedical discourse that addressed the same concerns but used different methods or models to explain malfunctions. *Hanbang* traditions, for example, had terms for ailments related to the pains associated with menstruation, menstrual irregularity, morning sickness, etc. And, in the case of *taeha*, it is clear that biomedical practitioners occasionally incorporated older terms or concepts suggestive of *hanbang*. One physician argued that a consequence of amenorrhea, besides biomedical explanations of abdominal aches, was the release of blood in other parts of the body, such as the nasal passages or gums, this being called *taesang wŏlgyŏng* (menoplania).[33]

One notion that emerged in *ŭisaeng* discussions that did not exist in Western gynecological thinking was *naeng* ("cold"), which, while attributable to older concepts of women's ailments, nonetheless fit in with biomedical notions of *puinbyŏng*. In print media, *naeng* was sometimes used interchangeably with *taeha*.[34] It was thought that the cold climate of winter months brought about more secretions. But *naeng* also referred in a classical sense to a state of the body when it lacked *yŏl* ("heat"), and thus signaled an imbalance affecting circulation.[35] Cho Hŏnyŏng, a scholar who studied *hanbang* independently, sold medicines based on Sino-classical medical prescriptions, and took a leading role in the *hanbang* revival movement of the 1930s, explained that those with *taeha* suffered from cold hands and feet and felt a cold sensation in their lower abdominal regions.[36] The purpose of countermeasures would be to keep those areas warm. Even physicians trained in biomedicine advised similar preventives. Cold weather and failure to keep the abdominal area sufficiently warm were thought to create more congestion, which could either incite inflammation of normal mucus or worsen existing inflammations.[37] The wearing of adequate clothing, lying under covers, and carrying a portable heating pad were encouraged.

The association between *puinbyŏng* and fertility was further made clear in attempts to synthesize biomedicine with older understandings of female bodies and ailments. Cho Hŏnyŏng generally situated biomedicine in opposition, yet complementary, to traditional medicine. Regarding *puinbyŏng*, he sought to clarify confusion around a constellation of notions surrounding cold ("*han*" and "*naeng*") and heat ("*hwa*" and "*yŏl*") that was common to both biomedical and *hanbang* traditions. Cho acknowledged the physiology of women's menstrual cycles and potential infections. He also recognized *hwabyŏng* as attributable to physiological factors, including mental stress.[38] "*Hwa*," he wrote, may not be due to excess *yŏl* in the body, and suggested prescriptions that were not geared toward attenuating one's bodily *yŏl*. Moreover, Cho warned his readers that some female patients could have "*hwa*" and "*naeng*" at the same time. To complicate matters, "*naeng*" might not be due to "*han*," so to treat it with "*yŏl*" would do harm. In short, it was imperative for the physician to determine the exact cause of the ailment (which could include a biomedical diagnosis), and if the ailment was due to bad blood, deficiencies in yin or yang, weaknesses in the visceral functions (according to Sino-classical medical theory), or overall weakness, then *hanbang* prescriptions could be effective.[39] His gynecological text *Puinbyŏng ch'iryobŏp* (Treating *puinbyŏng*, 1941) included a final chapter on how to treat ailments with a biomedical diagnosis such as hysteria and endometrial infections with *hanbang*.

IN SEARCH OF RELIEF

Although physicians in their reports or in print media often commented critically on women's efforts to seek solutions for their ailments with the intent to condemn the persistence of customs and health-related practices they deemed harmful or even barbaric, such accounts underline that women, for better or worse, actively sought relief by utilizing as many of the various forms of treatments and techniques as were available to them. The cases of female gynecological patients in hospitals, physicians asserted, were disgraceful. Such patients had often sought treatment for years, and only after failing to find relief through a myriad of evil practices such as acupuncture, moxibustion, or the singeing of flesh, did they seek treatment in the new hospitals.[40] That infertility was the overwhelming concern of these women was noted by Hall when she wrote that women's medical mission hospitals were "appealed to by a comparatively greater number of patients in Korea with relative sterility than at home."[41] Missionary physician Mary Stewart concurred, noting how the imperative for male progeny in Korean families—the successful carrying, delivering, and rearing of sons past the dangers of infancy—motivated women to seek medical help from hospitals. "Sterility is the source of great trouble in the Korean home. If no son is born the husband takes another wife; but upon consulting the doctor in a large majority of cases, after a month or so of care, pregnancy is reported. The news spread therefore our gynecological clinic reached nearly 2000 this last year."[42]

Even twenty-five years later in 1940, Dr. Pyŏn Ingi in Pyongyang noted that the family and the continuation of one's lineage were deemed among the most important things for Koreans, more so than in other countries. This created a culture where nothing was more precious or meaningful than the bearing of children, especially sons. The beauty of family (*kajŏng mi*) would be impossible without children, he continued, and a woman's childlessness, in the form of failure to conceive or carry to term, was a major concern of women who feared bringing ruin to the family.[43] The scandalous 1928 murder trial of a twenty-one-year-old married woman who stole and inadvertently killed a baby highlighted the tragic plight of childlessness for women in colonial Korea.[44] Yang Hyŏna's analysis of jurisprudence during the colonial period argues that changes in family law, which required every household be based on the conjugal unit and have a biological male descendant to succeed family-headship, institutionalized a family system even more patriarchal than in the Chosŏn dynasty.[45]

A major factor of women's infertility arose from complications that emerged from childbearing. At a time when most women gave birth at home, childbearing was especially dangerous, as many mothers injured their birth canal or peritoneum, developed infections or suffered a prolapsed uterus, which subsequently made it difficult for them to conceive or carry to term.[46] That a prolapsed uterus was a frequent enough occurrence to be of great concern is illustrated in fictional works of the time such as Kang Kyŏngae's short story, "Underground Village" (*Chiha ch'on*, 1936), in which the mother of the main character suffered from this ailment upon resuming work in the fields immediately after childbirth.[47] The condition usually resulted from inadequate postpartum care, particularly in women's lack of rest after delivery before the uterus had returned to its original size, and while its supporting ligaments remained stretched and loose. Another factor was excess stress on the uterus from multiple and frequent pregnancies.[48]

The enlarged uterus then protruded outside of the body, a condition that was unfortunately worsened in Korea by a common folk treatment— the burning off of the protrusion—practiced by itinerant female healers who earned scathing critiques from physicians for treating afflicted women with needles and burning metal.[49] The treatment sometimes resulted in a vesico-vaginal or recto-vaginal fistula, a painful and shameful condition, where the injury healed improperly so that the vagina and bladder or rectum became connected, plaguing women with the discomfort and embarrassment of a constant discharge of urine or feces as well as complicating conception and childbearing. It was possible to treat this condition, and Hall remarked that with proper surgical treatment some of her cases resulted in the fortunate birth of a child.[50] This helps account for the growing number of gynecological cases missionaries noted. Many of these cases were likely related to prolapsed uteruses or fistulas, as a 1917 mission report noted, "As a rule, of course, [gynecological cases] require operations or medicine or both. . . . Many are relieved not only of pain and other unpleasant symptoms but of their barrenness as well and often return to express their gratitude in different ways."[51] This faith that mission women's hospitals could successfully treat women's infertility drew increasing numbers of women in search of relief. Mary Stewart noted that the majority of receipts in dispensaries and returning visits to mission women's hospitals come from gynecological cases.[52] Statistics for female patients who visited the GGK provincial hospitals in 1930 present similar findings—the number-one reason why women visited the hospital was for urinary-reproductive ailments.[53] Physicians writing in popular journals also encouraged women to seek medical treatment. Hŏ Sin reminded his readers that it was possible to conceive even with a displaced uterus, damaged ovaries, or *puinbyŏng* in the hands of a reputable gynecologist.[54]

Missionary physician Mary Cutler at the Woman's Hospital of Extended Grace in Pyongyang described in 1918 what she saw as the main problems in women's health in Korea: "the superstitions to be overcome, rare diseases and anomalies in anatomical structures seen. Often that which ought to be seen or felt is congenitally wanting, or has been mechanically obliterated, obscured, or obstructed, usually by burning, and is the cause behind much of our gynecological and obstetrical work."[55] The reality was that childbearing for most parts of the world, including Korea, remained dangerous in the early twentieth century.[56] There was little physicians could do for a new mother with peritonitis or other septic infections before the mass production and use of sulfa drugs and antibiotics. Other complications in addition to the prolapsed uterus and fistulas, included toxemia, whether by eclampsia (a condition where protein collects in the urine, body tissues swell, and blood pressure rises, leading to convulsions, coma, and even death if untreated), tissues of the fetus entering and thus poisoning the mother's bloodstream, or hemorrhage with little recourse without blood transfusions. Congenital defects (small pelvis) or damage to the pelvic bones by nutritional deficiency diseases such as rickets, also complicated delivery for many women.[57] As a former gynecologist later recalled, the top three causes of maternal mortality during the colonial period were pre-eclampsia, infections, and hemorrhage.[58] Even should a woman survive childbirth, she usually suffered from other long-term damage to her body. Without access to proper medical care and facilities, and with little recourse besides caesarean or forceps delivery even in hospitals, women were apt to seek folk or homemade treatments for their ailments.

In this context, proper postpartum care was even more critical not only for the well-being of a parturient mother but also to protect her future reproductive health. While missionary physicians were optimistic that their surgical procedures could rectify anatomical anomalies and help a woman conceive, other physicians disagreed, arguing that once a fistula fully formed, it was too late. They also claimed that improper sexual relations, childbearing techniques, and postpartum care produced the multitude of infections and injuries that brought on *puinbyŏng* and infertility. Korean physicians castigated what they called unhygienic practices such as the immediate return of women to household chores after childbearing. They desired police regulation to restrict the activity of itinerant healers, along with better enforcement of unlicensed "midwives," whose lack of education and disinfecting techniques were blamed for producing infections leading to *puinbyŏng* or the dreaded puerperal fever that usually killed new mothers.[59] Gynecologist Yun T'aegwŏn recalled an especially horrifying case he had of a macerated fetus and a woman near death due to mishandling by an incompetent itinerant healer.[60]

Korean women sought medications and relief from ailments in terms with which they were familiar. In this way, *puinbyŏng* offers a fascinating example of the ways modern practices and knowledge of the body and medicine re-appropriated older traditions in ways that Theodore Jun Yoo calls a "palimpsest of memory: inscriptions of new understandings, which partially effaced yet never fully erased older ones."[61] *Taeha* and *naeng* (likely referring to leukorrhea in this context), for example, were noted by physicians as common complaints among their patients and advice seekers. Kim Sŏkhwan, a physician at the teaching hospital of Keijō Imperial University, recalled one of his female patients who was swindled by an itinerant saleswoman-healer who sold her a silver needle on the claims it would cure her of *naeng*.[62] A columnist for a family health newspaper column, he asserted that the majority of requests he received were for advice in dealing with *taeha*.[63]

Attempts at self-treatment and self-medication were abetted by the new pharmaceutical industry. Pharmaceuticals were the most advertised products in colonial Korea.[64] While at present there is little information on the level of consumption of these products or their sales figures, the fact that there were many different kinds of medications, developed by both Korean and Japanese pharmaceutical companies, sold throughout the colonial period attests to the presence of a steady demand for medicines to treat afflictions—especially *puinbyŏng*—in the privacy of one's own home. Studies on medical consumption behavior of the general Korean population in the colonial period indicate that folk remedies and self-medication were the most popular forms of therapies.[65] A 1929 survey of Korean residents in the Suwŏn District, for example, recounts how one woman sought the services of a shaman instead of a hospital to treat her daughter's *puinbyŏng*. The same survey also notes that a low-level patrol officer sought to self-treat a long-term case of syphilis with patent medicines.[66]

In her analysis of patent medicines in Meiji and Taishō Japan, Susan Burns demonstrates how the visual iconography and narratives of advertising intersected with the formation of modern subjectivities.[67] Advertisements in colonial Korea likewise could channel consumer choices by giving form to new cultural imaginings of idealized lifestyles and shaping expectations and aspirations.[68] Advertisements helped shape the experience of being sick by not only providing medical information to readers, but also instructing them how to be sick, playing on their personal desires and making attractive an alternative lifestyle (one of health, or in this case, of bearing children).

In colonial Korea, patent medicine advertisements deployed medical understandings of both older and biomedical traditions. They appealed because they evoked familiar explanations of women's ailments such as cold limbs and the need to improve circulation (which ambiguously could refer to either physiological circulation of the bloodstream or metaphysical circulation of in *hanbang* terms), through means such as warming of the uterus, while also promising efficacy backed by scientific authority. For example, Megumi no Tama ("Jewel of Benevolence") claimed to control the female hormones in order to treat infertility, menstrual disorders, *naengbyŏng*, and pelvic inflammations, among other symptoms, and also promised the restoration of feminine beauty as highlighted by the illustration of two young demure women in Korean-style *hanbok*.[69] Another medication that conjured associations with the new field of endocrinology was Obasumon, which claimed that its main ingredient was a female hormone extracted from animals. This was to invigorate the blood and be highly effective for problems related to menstruation, infertility, frigidity, and nervous disorders.[70] The list of symptoms for which Obasumon was indicated included menstrual irregularity and early menopause. Other similar products included Obahorumon, Oophormin, and Estemon, the latter promising to resolve hormonal secretions.[71]

Early patent medicines based on *hanbang* prescriptions to treat women's disease and infertility also were popular. These included T'aeyangjogyŏnghwan ("Pill of Fetal Nourishment and Menstrual Regulation") in the 1910s, which was one of the best sellers of its company. It claimed efficacy in treating menstrual irregularity, *taeha*, and infertility.[72] Paekpohwan ("Pill of Nourishment with One Hundred Ingredients)," another popular product, discussed infertility and uterine diseases in its advertisements, "urging women to consume the pill instead of praying for a baby in a Buddhist temple."[73] Chogyŏngchongokhwan ("Jewel Pill of Menstrual Regulation") was a mainstay of its company.[74] Misinhwan ("Pill of Beautiful Spirit") offered treatment as effective as surgery to recover youth, beauty, and marital harmony using the latest *puinbyŏng* therapies to treat *taehajŭng*, regulate the menses, improve circulation, and heat the body.[75] Ads for these products featured illustrations of mother and child and photographs of the many babies conceived by women consumers who faithfully took the medications.[76]

Advertisements for these projects also served as a means to convey medical knowledge about women's bodies and reproductive health to potential consumers. For example, ads for Inochi No Haha ("Mother of Life") appeared over an extended period of time and in large spreads, functioning similarly to today's infomercials.[77] At times, its advertise-ments appeared in newspapers disguised as informative articles with titles such as, "Simple self-remedies to take at home for *puinbyŏng*, which takes your beauty and prevents you from having children." "Whose fault is it that one cannot have a child?" "Infertility is all due to *puinbyŏng*." "How can I resolve this by self-treatment at home?" "Comparing West-ern and Eastern *puinbyŏng* remedies."[78] At other times, the promotions for "Mother of Life" appeared as typical advertisements, with images and a brief list of the symptoms that could be remedied. It was advertised at times with another product, Oginaku, which appears to have been some form of hormonal injection.

The advertising for "Mother of Life" played up a woman's fears that she would lose her beauty, her body would become sick, her face would show fatigue, she would lose harmonious relations with her husband, and fail to conceive or carry babies to term. She was advised to look for a whole array of symptoms: headaches, insomnia, indigestion, weak-ness, itchy or swollen genitalia, constipation, urination urges, leukor-rhea, menstrual irregularity or pain, cold limbs, tightness in the chest, hysteria, and feelings of jealousy or agitation. Consumers were to record their symptoms in detail and send them in along with the amount of medication desired, upon which the company would mail the appropri-ate medication and a free booklet on *puinbyŏng*. The medication could be taken before marriage, during pregnancy, and after delivery to for-tify the maternal body. Advertisements used images of mothers with child(ren) to convey the message that the ultimate purpose of "Mother of Life" was to prepare the body for producing babies or to resolve infertil-ity issues. They also used images of a male physician in a white lab coat and spectacles to stress the product's scientific authority, claiming it was backed by over thirty years of research and experience at an unnamed university hospital. Like other patent medicines in this period, promot-ers were vague at best about its active ingredients and how it functioned. "Mother of Life," it appeared, borrowed from both biomedical and *han-bang* principles to improve circulation, expel toxins, warm the uterus, and heal areas of pain. The major selling point of these medications was their claim to successfully address *puinbyŏng* and, thereby, ensure women's fertility.

"LIMITING BIRTH" AND THE
POLITICS OF BIRTH CONTROL

Despite women's apparent determination to achieve successful pregnancies, knowledge of the physiology of reproduction and medications that aimed to regulate women's menstrual cycles by stimulating the shedding of the uterine lining could also be, and in fact were, wielded by women to terminate pregnancies. In 1922, a Japanese teacher at a public common school in Chŏngju died from complications after trying to stimulate a miscarriage with medications when seven months pregnant.[79] Another woman died from ingesting hair dye because she had heard it was "nice" for menstrual irregularity.[80] Recourse to medications was portrayed in the 1931 short story "Miscarriage" (*Yusan*), in which the protagonist is advised by her husband to end her unwanted pregnancy in this way.[81] Popular representations of the availability of such medications were satirized in a fictional roundtable printed in the journal *Pyŏlgŏngon* in which the physician character conflated the abortifacients he prescribes to female students for their unwanted pregnancies with birth control.[82]

Korea's criminal code under the GGK made punishable any abortion or abortion-related activity and the GGK began to prosecute women for procuring abortions.[83] Yet, despite the threat of punishment, abortions and intentional miscarriages (included under the broad category of abortion called *t'at'ae* or "falling of the fetus") occurred on a relatively frequent basis. Newspapers reported women falling from high precipices or ingesting large quantities of lye or soy sauce in the hopes of ending pregnancies. The GGK published the number of prosecuted abortion cases in its annual statistical yearbook, although these figures are ambiguous for it is not clear whether the defendants were women who procured abortions, persons who performed abortions, or others whose physical assault inadvertently induced a miscarriage (the latter charge hearkening back to earlier forms of criminalization of abortion in Chosŏn law).

The criminalization of abortion has been understood as part of a larger strategy for population growth to produce the human resources necessary for Japanese imperialist expansion.[84] The GGK's promotion of a modern midwifery system was in part to prevent infanticide and abortions, as were "loving and protecting the child" infant welfare events and the *kasa* (domestic science) curriculum in girls' higher common schools for young women to learn the physiology of pregnancy and proper child-rearing techniques. The GGK also implemented what Jin-kyung Park calls "corporeal colonialism," deliberate investigations and interventions focused on the Korean female body to manage the Korean population.[85] Medical research on women's reproductive systems and procreative abilities, licensing of prostitution and control of sexually transmitted diseases, and condemnation of the custom of early marriage all were part of a regime to enhance Korean women's fertility.[86]

The goal of increasing numbers, however, contended with other anxieties, such as the "population problem" based on Malthusian theories, which questioned the desirability of a large population that might exceed resources, and notions of civilization based on healthy and well-educated citizens.[87] These contradictory impulses created the possibility for Koreans to advocate for the means to control, or even stop, reproduction. In other words, while the overarching objective of the GGK's biopolitics was to increase the population by focusing primarily on female reproduction, the GGK also aimed to take measures that it perceived would improve the *quality* of that population. This invited not only the overhaul of the public health and medical services discussed in the previous two chapters but also discussions of women's physiology and reproductive health on which proponents of birth control could base their position.[88]

While abortion was criminalized, there was no absolute censorship of birth control in Japan.[89] Restrictions on advertising were placed on products or substances that specified their use as contraceptives, but their limited sale (by mail) and utilization otherwise were permitted. Sources indicate that indeed some contraceptive methods were available and known to at least a segment of the Korean population—mainly urban and educated, especially if they had studied abroad in Japan. The methods were explained in a surprisingly detailed manner in print media, and while descriptions of certain forms of contraceptives could not be publicized, knowledge of the physiology of conception did circulate. Physician authors explained the female reproductive system including the processes of ovulation, in medical terms. They introduced different methods of birth control (condom, pessary, sponge or other suppositories, drugs, washing or douching, X-ray, surgery, rhythm method), weighing their merits and demerits.[90] Female readers, could learn to calculate the days they were not ovulating as a crude form of contraception (the rhythm method), a technique that was commonly used in Japan.[91] An T'aeyun's oral interviews with women who lived through this period reveal that female students who learned about the method during the colonial period practiced it.[92] Furthermore, knowledge on the viability of sperm in an acidic or alkaline environment, or the efficacy of washing immediately after coitus, added information to the repertoire of knowledge of a woman who wanted to control her reproduction.

Discussion of birth control was not limited to physicians. Pak Hojin, an active member of the women's organization *Kŭnuhoe*, defined a woman-centered position on birth control that emerged from the beginning of birth control discussions. To her, Korean women lived in a constant state of pregnancy, with short periods of recovery between deliveries. Child-rearing, moreover, sapped the energy and efforts of women. She argued in 1930 that birth control in Korea would allow women to develop and display their talents and personalities as people.[93] A few years later, artist Chang Ch'ŏnyŏng expressed support for birth control as well, admitting that caring for her child was keeping her from her art.[94] And Na Hyesŏk, the well-known literary figure who was central to debates about the New Woman in colonial Korea, advocated for birth control in "experimental" or "trial marriages" so as not to laden the relationship with children in case of failure.[95]

One of the more articulate woman-centered positions supporting birth control was that of Yun Sŏngsang, one of the first female reporters for *Chosŏn ilbo* and a member of *Kŭnuhoe*.[96] She summarized the various arguments against birth control—it was unethical, encouraged extramarital affairs and the dissolution of marriages, prevented the birth of potential geniuses, and caused *puinbyŏng* or infertility—and countered them one by one. For Yun, the fundamental issue was that women's desire for birth control was natural, even an instinct, if latent. Quoting directly from Margaret Sanger, she explained that women's desire for family limitation—which could be horrifically manifested in infanticide, abortion, and abandoned children—might stem from economic oppression or the desire for freedom. Yun rejected the notion of women being mere reproductive vessels owned by men. She argued for the practice of birth control in the Korean context to ensure there were enough resources to raise children properly, hinting at Korea's poor economic state. She also cited the protection of maternal health, for women were equal to men as members of society. Both men and women had to work together to develop society, but having too many children taxed women's bodies, thus preventing their full participation.

In the end, however, the prevailing discourse on birth control in colonial Korea was not about women's self-determination or liberation.[97] Rather, it was about reproducing in a manner that benefited one's society, nation, or empire. The terms used to translate birth control in colonial Korea were *sana chehan* ("limiting birth") and *sana chojŏl* ("adjusting/controlling birth") with the former being more commonly used. Implicit in "adjusting" or "controlling" was the ability to choose when and how many children one would bear. "Limiting" suggests the reduction in the number of births, which was controversial in light of the GGK's population policy. It was not about *not* having children altogether. In a 1930 survey, notable female figures including Kim Wŏnju, Na Hyesŏk, Hŏ Yŏngsuk, and Hwang Sindŏk were asked whether they practiced birth control as well as how many children they desired, thus linking, not severing, birth control and reproduction.[98] As Yun Sŏngsang clarified, birth control was not about preventing births; it was about preventing excessive births and raising well those children who were born. And, as noted by Pae Sŏngnyong, it was something women could do with the new products, medical services, and knowledge of their bodies now available: "Limiting birth is the avoidance of conception by women themselves through technological means."[99]

The voices of Korean women of the early 1930s, however, were displaced as Japan's war with China led to an increasingly militarized society. Greater restrictions were placed on birth control activities and discussions became dominated by male intellectuals and physicians. Women-centered positions on birth control were quickly pushed aside in favor of neo-Malthusian connections between overpopulation and poverty, state-sponsored protections of maternal and children's health, and support for medicalized eugenics.[100] While women-centered positions may have been expressed, they were articulated in terms that directly connected them to women's roles as mothers and guardians of the next generation. For example, Christian women leaders in female education such as Pak Killae may have disapproved of pronatalist policies in Italy and Germany for treating women too much like "tools of reproduction (*saengsan kigu*)." Cho Hyŏngyŏng, who had studied abroad in Japan and was employed as a teacher at Ewha may have called for birth control partly for the sake of improving women's status. But both Pak and Cho were involved with the women's journal *Yŏron* (Pak on the writing staff and Cho as one of its founders), which aimed at "family improvement" through education, and Cho, in particular, framed the improvement of women's status through birth control as not for women's own sake but to allow them more time to cultivate themselves to be better at their roles as mothers and wives.[101]

Gynecological discussions on *puinbyŏng* that warned against the dangers of improper postpartum care and the stress posed by multiple births spilled over into debates on birth control as well. Like Chosŏn period gynecological concerns regarding women's fertility, the attention on women's menstruation and pregnancy in colonial Korean gynecology were directed toward the prevention of infertility arising from potential complications. Gynecology separated itself from obstetrics as the colonial medical system positioned midwives as the primary providers of childbirth services, with physicians expected to step in only for complicated deliveries or "abnormal" pregnancies. To avoid complications and lessen infant morbidity, physicians recommended delaying childbirth and spacing children, the very premises on which birth control proponents based their arguments.

At the heart of discussions of *puinbyŏng* and birth control was anxiety about the next generation, whether it was to meet the desires of the Korean patriarchal family, visions of healthy Christian families, or the needs of nationalist or imperialist mobilizations. While some articulated the fear that reduction of the population would lead to race suicide (by depriving society of the potential birth of future leaders), these were countered by eugenics-oriented reasoning.[102] It was asserted that society could improve by prohibiting the procreation of certain categories of the "unfit." This would allow families to save for or have enough financial and emotional resources to raise the "fit" as educated, productive members of society. The logic of eugenic thinking in colonial Korea also posited that having large numbers of children would inevitably produce some who were talentless, inferior, or impoverished.

Practicing birth control would, the argument continued, prevent their births.[103]

The term eugenics, *usaeng*, emerged in Korean print media in the early 1920s and was discussed along with new genetic knowledge starting in the latter 1920s. The concept was generally discussed in relation to marriage (choosing proper partners), and was heavily promoted in Korea by Yi Kapsu, a physician who had graduated from Keijō Medical College in 1920, studied in Germany and Japan, opened his own clinic, and later taught at the *kasa* department of Ewha Womans College and the Korean women's medical school.[104] In 1933, Yi along with other social reformers established the Korean Eugenics Association (*Chosŏn usaeng hyŏphoe*). According to its publication *Usaeng* (Eugenics), the rather illustrious membership roster included Yun Ch'iho, Yŏ Ŭnhyŏng, and Kim Hwallan. Their membership lent respectability to eugenics, paraded as science.[105]

In the Korean colonial context, the burgeoning field of gynecology and debates on birth control contributed to the construction of a womanhood that tied women to their biological and social functions as mothers and viewed their reproduction as meeting the needs of family, society, nation, and empire. Women's bodies were to function foremost in this reproductive role, and failure to do so was tragic (in the case of infertility) or abominable (in the case of choice). Women's reproductive health was so paramount that it touched most issues related to women's rights or activities. For example, the *Tonga ilbo* reported rumors that men were reluctant to marry women who worked at a particular silk-reeling factory in Japan as their harsh working conditions deteriorated the health of workers and left many of them sterile.[106] This was part of a larger discussion of the effect work had on women's health and fertility. Physician Pyŏn Sŏkhwa warned that women who stood or sat crouched all day experienced harm to their reproductive system.[107] Pressure placed on the pelvis and exhaustion could prevent the proper development of reproductive organs, bring on menstrual disorders, spontaneous miscarriage, early labor, or even sterility. This affected not only factory laborers but also office workers, bus girls, phone operators, students, and even musicians. Labor activists used similar medical reasoning in calls for improved working conditions with rests (including those during menstruation and breastfeeding) for women, again, to protect their reproductive health and the viability of the next generation. Female students were instructed to exercise—good for the body, good for the mind—but cautioned not to overexert themselves.

For this reason, women's health was critical, but not so much for the sake of their liberation, happiness, or well-being. While better opportunities may have opened to women in the form of new occupations in the growing health industry, medical technology allowed for some control over their reproduction, and higher living standards better enabled women to follow their pursuits; medical discourse on the whole marginalized women's health concerns unrelated to fertility. Physicians may have urged women not to assign harsh labor to their daughters-in-law so as to give them space and time to recover after childbirth, but again this was in the context of protecting their daughters-in-law from *puinbyŏng* and not for the sake of easing familial relations.[108] Diseases of the breasts, such as mastitis or breast cancer, were not included in the notion of *puinbyŏng*, while seemingly nongendered ailments, such as beriberi or anemia were, as they related to complicating pregnancy or the reproductive system. When asked what causes they would take if they were activists in women's movements, well-known Korean male figures listed education, rural issues, economics (encouraging thrift), production, and marriage.[109] Organizing around women's health issues did not occur much in this period.

Health of the Korean people, the dominant discourse asserted, began not with children but with pregnant women, in other words, their wombs.[110] Therefore, the focus of a woman's care was to be on her reproductive health for it would critically shape her unborn child. If her physical and mental state affected the development of her fetus and his or her future capabilities after birth as proponents of *t'aegyo* ("fetal education," a form of practices related to prenatal care, and the character, intellectual, and mental development of the unborn child) would argue, a woman was to learn the latest health directives and employ proper medical services and products available to her, including the practice of "limiting birth."[111]

Nevertheless, as Frank Dikötter argues in regard to Republican China, gynecological texts and health manuals might have constructed women as the weaker sex by representing "menstruation as a pathological process," signaling female instability as women's mental and physical states were easily affected during menstruation. But women were also "relatively autonomous individuals who were given a responsibility over their own bodily secretions for the sake of reproductive health."[112] While the imperative to reproduce remained constant, as demonstrated in this chapter, women also took the initiative to make reproductive choices and advocate for their personal interests, employing the many options that became available. There are indications that coming to know their bodies, the physiology of their menstruation, and probable causes of infertility or "women's disease" enabled and empowered women to understand why their bodies behaved the way they did and to seek treatment suited to their personal circumstances.

Increased knowledge also empowered women to take preventive measures to secure healthier lives, such as to demand venereal testing from their prospective spouses or birth control to limit physical stress and harm to their bodies. Even women whose bodies were not conventionally seen as reproductive and marginalized from the Wise Mother, Good Wife idealization, such as *kisaeng*, sought to protect their health by sharing knowledge among themselves about their gynecological health.[113] And if women lacked the means or inclination to visit a hospital, they sought alternate methods including folk remedies and patent medicines. An attraction of such medications was that they could help avoid the embarrassment women faced in addressing their very personal and private afflictions. "Treat yourself in the privacy or secrecy of your home." "No one needs to know." Also important in advertising appeals was women's concern to achieve feminine beauty, family harmony, and, reading between the lines, sexual pleasure.

EPILOGUE

In 1938, female physician Hŏ Yŏngsuk started what she claimed was Korea's first maternity clinic. In so doing, she hoped to prevent maternal mortality and injuries sustained during delivery as well as ensure the welfare of infants. For Hŏ, the ideal maternity clinic differed from other hospitals, including specialized gynecological hospitals, in the care of female patients. It was to be a space devoted solely to the health needs of birthing mothers and their newborns. More importantly, the practices of the new clinic were to be based on the physiological knowledge of childbearing and techniques of modern obstetrics that Hŏ had cultivated during her study abroad at the Red Cross maternity clinic in Tokyo in the mid-1930s. A maternity clinic done well, she noted, could save two lives. Echoing turn-of-the-twentieth-century logic in public health discussions that measured civilization by the health of the population, Hŏ asserted that the ways in which the health of parturient mothers was tended would reflect not only the happiness of the women involved but also the level of civilization their society had attained.[1]

It is not surprising that Hŏ Yŏngsuk, a female physician with children of her own and reformist inclinations, would start a maternity clinic. In many ways, she epitomized the expectations of Korean women in the field of medicine and how far they had come. As described in the preceding chapters, while foreign missionaries in the 1880s and 1890s faced difficulties recruiting female pupils to their schools, not to mention the challenge of retaining suitable medical assistants in their clinics, by the 1930s many Korean women aspired to, and indeed acquired, formal education as well as the professional skills befitting a modern era. Hŏ Yŏngsuk represented many "firsts" in the history of women and medicine in Korea—the first Korean graduate of Tokyo Women's Medical College, the first Korean woman to receive a physician's license from the GGK, the first Korean woman to open a private medical practice. She wrote a long-running series on women's and family health for the vernacular daily newspaper the *Tonga ilbo* in the mid-1920s. While not actively involved in its founding, she moderated the 1928 inaugural assembly of the organizers of Korea's first women's medical school, the Korean Women's Medical Training Institute.[2] The general trend of the time supported and encouraged the education and practice of women in medicine. Yet, as Hŏ herself wrote, her maternity clinic transpired only after years of effort on her part, opening nearly a decade after she quit her private medical practice.

Understanding why it took so long requires situating Hŏ within the medical and gendered context of colonial Korean society. Earlier in a 1930 survey conducted by the journal *Pyŏlgŏngon*, Hŏ had expressed dissatisfaction with herself, stating that were she a man, she would not marry a woman like herself.[3] She admitted that she was highly educated, possessing medical skills with the ability and desire to do much for the women in her country, but lamented that she nonetheless was unable to do much. While such comments and assertions of having many embarrassing flaws suggest a humility that was culturally common in the rhetoric of her time, they also reveal frustrations Hŏ attempted to mask over not being able to work. Piecing together different statements she made publicly throughout the 1920s and 1930s, one can deduce that her domestic responsibilities and duties to her household and children were the primary reasons she did not actively practice medicine. One of her contemporaries expressed regret that Hŏ, despite her tremendous skills, remained basically the personal physician of her husband, the famed literary figure Yi Kwangsu.[4]

Hŏ's ultimate success in establishing her maternity clinic occurred at a time when anxieties over poor maternal health and infant mortality rates ran high in Korean society and Japanese officialdom, fueling public and popular support for endeavors such as hers. The year of its founding coincided with the escalation of the Japanese military aggression in

China that stoked official urgency to mobilize all subjects in support of Japan's imperialist ambitions.[5] As wartime exigencies "transformed the population problem to that of a lack," the Korean colonial population was reconfigured as one that "should be healthy, reproductive, and long lived."[6] This, according to Takashi Fujitani, produced the contradiction in Japan's post-1937 racial and welfare policies that folded colonial subjects within the larger category of the "Japanese" in new ways, tantalizing with promises of future (but deferred and ultimately not granted) political and social citizenship and rights at the same time it extracted human resources and labor from colonial subjects' bodies (for example, as soldiers). The new Ministry of Health and Welfare in the Japanese metropole was established in 1938 for the purpose of promoting the welfare and cultivation of human resources. The GGK's Bureau of Health and Welfare, established a few years later in 1941, similarly addressed issues ranging from "the improvement of physical strength, maternity, infants and young children, public health issues, food and water, labor and unemployment, social and medical relief."[7]

The convergence of the GGK's mobilization efforts, the establishment of Ho's maternity clinic, the accreditation of the Keijō Women's Medical Training Institute as a professional school (renamed the Keijō Women's Medical College), and the removal of foreign missionaries created new conditions for women's experiences in health and medicine. The GGK's efforts to mobilize medical personnel and resources led to shifts in health administration and orientation, such as the expanding interest in medicinal properties of *hanbang* prescriptions and the reduction in the time required for the training of nurses. Keijō Women's Medical College may have achieved accreditation with the timely and generous donation bequeathed by Kim Chongik in 1938, but the GGK, which had previously shown little interest in Korean women's medical schools, soon after began contributing 200,000 yen annually to support the increasing number of Japanese female students who were coming to Korea to study.[8] The hostile environment toward, and eventual forcible removal of, Christian missionaries resulted in the transfer of the administration of medical facilities, including infant welfare clinics, to Korean hands, female as well as male.

With the increasingly pronatalist agenda, Japanese authorities turned their attention to improving the state of maternal health and infant welfare, prohibiting birth control and other threats to female reproduction, and promoting procreation both in the metropole and the colonies. The arrest of famed Japanese birth control advocate Ishimoto Shizue in December 1937 precipitated the closure of birth control clinics in Japan.[9] In Korea, discussions of birth control, which in the 1920s and 1930s had been framed around issues of maternal health and women's desires, now ceased to appear in the print media. Slogans such as "Give birth and multiply" and "Five children per woman," became common.[10] The GGK's Bureau of Health and Welfare aimed to increase the population by encouraging marriage and reproduction. It made plans for prenatal facilities and milk services though those failed to materialize to any real extent.[11] Efforts to encourage women to have children included increasing food rations to expectant mothers and offering awards to mothers with more than ten surviving children.[12] Among conditions for an award were that all children were to be over the age of six, all were to be healthy, and the families were determined to be of good character.[13]

One aspect of Japanese pronatalist policies that had a lasting impact on Korea was the growing emphasis on eugenics. The Ministry of Health and Welfare organized a Eugenics Section with a Racial Hygiene Study Group, and promulgated the 1940 National Eugenics Law (*Kokumin yōsei hō*), often known as the sterilization law, modeled upon a German racial hygiene law, which "allowed the government to order the sterilization of people with hereditary illnesses, . . . [including] hereditary mental illness, hereditary mental deficiency, severe and malignant hereditary personality disorder, severe and malignant hereditary physical ailment, and severe hereditary deformity."[14] The sterilization law was put into effect in 1941 in Japan with plans for extension to Korea a few years later but the exigencies of war resulted in its limited enforcement.[15] In Korea, only male patients with Hansen's disease (leprosy) in the colonial government's isolation facility at Sorokdo were affected. The sterilization law also reflected pronatalist dimensions in eugenics practice in the Japanese empire by restricting the sterilization of young persons found clear of suspect diseases in required examinations.[16] This promoted, or at least prevented attempts to obstruct or block, the reproduction of the "fit," befitting the literal meaning of eugenics or, as translated in Korean, *usaeng* (優生), "birthing of the superior" or "well-born."[17] Pre-1938 discussions in Korean print media of sterilization as a method of birth control were no longer an option, further limiting the choices Koreans could make in determining their own reproductive lives.

Nevertheless, the ready acceptance of the logic of eugenics persisted post-1945 and shaped general discussions around women's birth control. For example, Yi Kapsu of the Korean Eugenics Society, active during the colonial period, was appointed vice-director of South Korea's first Ministry of Public Health in the postliberation era and was integral to efforts to introduce a eugenics bill in the 1960s.[18] The Korean Eugenics Society itself was resurrected in 1946 as the "Korean National Eugenics Association" (*Hanguk minjok usaeng hyŏphoe*), which advocated for eugenics legislation. Although its efforts did not produce results in the 1960s, eugenic notions were incorporated into the 1973 Mother and Child Health Act (*Moja pogŏnbŏp*), which effectively replaced the former colonial prohibitions against abortion, allowing it in cases for stipulated reasons including suspected hereditary disease or illness, both mental and physical, and when the health of a mother and/or child was endangered.[19] The overlap between eugenics and maternal-infant welfare in reproductive politics becomes clearer when looking at slogans in post-1945 family planning campaigns that framed eugenics as maternal and infant health concerns.[20]

While there are some elements that persist, one cannot argue for seamless continuity from the colonial period into the present regarding birth control or other reproductive practices. The changed sociopolitical environment after liberation produced a new cadre of leaders who had the resources, desire, and organization to establish a family planning campaign that has been touted as one of the most successful in the world. What I want to suggest, rather, is that a key feature of reproductive and medical practice in Korea today is the continued purported notion that women's bodies are to function foremost in their reproductive and child-rearing capacities as mothers, often to meet national or familial goals.[21] The South Korean state at both the national and local levels continues to seek to mobilize women's wombs for state purposes, whether to reduce the population (as in the 1960s) or increase it (today). These efforts are buttressed by developments in medical practice, the pharmaceutical industry, and consumer markets.[22]

Returning to Hŏ Yŏngsuk, her story suggests the ways women, their bodies, and their health embodied the contradictions in Korea's attempts to prevent, treat, and manage disease and ailments in the early twentieth century. Calls to improve the health of the populace and the status of women arose from the same modernist visions that altered conceptions of the population on the whole and women in particular in relation to their potential contributions to larger social units such as the state. As such, efforts to develop a modern health regime were aimed at preparing women for their newly defined roles in reformist, Christian, and nation- or empire-building projects. Yet these "sanitizing" engagements intersected with the material conditions of Korean society as well as Japanese imperialist, Korean nationalist, patriarchal, paternalistic, and Christian evangelizing imperatives. They thus produced uneven developments and imparted a mixed legacy for postcolonial Korea. Moreover, the contours of these projects were gendered, shaping not only new expectations for women's roles and work, but also the ways women were situated in, and experienced, medical modernization.

The resulting reorganization of public sanitation, education, medical services, therapeutics, and health behavior relied in part on the reformation of Korean women who were now cast as reproducers and health care providers of a newly conceived populace, entrusted to guard the health of themselves, their families, and other women and children. Women stood out in the medical landscape, perhaps not so much in numbers but as targets of health education, reform measures, policy making, pharmaceutical advertisements, and medical research. Yet many women struggled to gain genuine recognition or support for their medical participation. This would not change as long as women in medicine remained tied to their gendered roles—responsible for the care of women's reproductive health and children. Figures from a 1986 report by the Korean Women's Medical Association (*Hanguk yŏja ŭisahoe*) indicate that female physicians still were overwhelmingly concentrated in the specialties of pediatrics and obstetrics-gynecology.[23]

Nevertheless, the construction of women as maternal bodies in both reproducing and nurturing roles was not absolute, and other conceptualizations of womanhood continually challenged the focus on motherhood, producing moments of tension. Women pursued recognition in their medical careers and rejected condescending treatment. They sought decision making in their reproductive health and child-rearing roles for considerations other than God, family, nation, or empire. They ignored prohibitions on birth control and abortion, seeking means to restrict the number of children they would have.[24] They demanded fertility treatments and reformulated traditions of prenatal care into their birthing practices. They asked physicians to conduct thorough physical examinations of their children at infant welfare clinics. In the end, even as Korean women had much to contend with, their energy and efforts shaped the story of modern medicine in Korea.

NOTES

INTRODUCTION

1. "Yŏ'in sŏngsim (A woman's sincerity)," *Cheguk sinmun*, May 19, 1899.
2. While girls' schools in the late nineteenth century enrolled students from a wide range of ages including those we today might construe as adults, "girl" will be used instead of "woman" as these schools offered only an elementary level of education at this time.
3. Korea's conclusion of a treaty with Japan that opened the ports of Inch'ŏn, Pusan, and Wŏnsan to trade and Japanese settlement in 1876 ushered in what has been called the "Open Ports Period." Other countries such as the United States and France concluded similar treaties with Korea in the 1880s.
4. When it appeared that the state would not fund a girls' school, the Ch'anyanghoe started the Sunsŏng Girls' School, which, like other private schools of the period, suffered from a lack of finances and administrative commitment. The last public record of this school was in 1905.
5. This is in contrast to rates of 30 percent and 47.4 percent, respectively, of the Korean male population who received primary education. Kim Puja, *Hakkyo pak ŭi Chosŏn yŏsŏngtŭl* [Korean women outside of school], trans. Cho Kyŏnghŭi and Kim Uja (Seoul: Ilchogak, 2005), 159.
6. Ch'ang Haeja, "Yŏhaksaeng ege ŭihak yŏngu rŭl kwŏngo" [Encouraging female students to medical study], *Taehan hŭnghakpo* 6 (1909).
7. Horace Allen, attendant physician of the royal hospital Chejungwŏn established in 1885, requested female medical assistants, noting the reluctance of female patients to be seen by male physicians.
8. This Training Institute underwent several changes in its history. In 1933, its name was changed to Keijō Women's Medical Training Institute. It achieved professional school status in 1938, becoming Keijō Women's Medical College (*Kyŏngsŏng yŏja ŭihak chŏnmun hakkyo*). After

liberation, its name was changed to Seoul Women's Medical School (Seoul *yŏja ŭigwa taehak*). As Sudo Medical School, it began to accept male students in 1957, evolving to a general college a decade later (Usŏk College) before its final incarnation as the College of Medicine at Korea University. Kil Chŏnghŭi, *Na ŭi chasŏjŏn* [My memoirs] (Seoul: Samho ch'ulp'ansa, 1981), 32–33.

9. Prior to this, graduates of the Training Institute were required to pass the physician licensing examination before being allowed to practice.

10. This definition of medicine comes from the online Merriam-Webster dictionary. http://www.merriam-webster.com/dictionary/medicine, accessed November 29, 2015.

11. The Yellow Emperor is the famed ancient Chinese emperor whose questions with his physician form the text of the *Inner Canon of the Yellow Emperor* (dates estimated between fifth c. BCE to second c. CE). The Chinese origin of official medicine in Korea remains a point of contention among scholars and practitioners today, but there is no question Korean kingdoms were exposed to and accommodated Chinese medical theory and techniques as part of a larger rubric of knowledge representing advanced civilization. See works such as Miki Sakae, *Chōsen igakkushi oyobi shippeishi* [History of Korean medicine and of disease in Korea] (Osaka, Japan: Shibun chuppansha, 1963); Kim Tujong, *Hanguk ŭihaksa chŏn* [History of Korean medicine] (Seoul: T'amgudang, 1966); and Sin Tongwŏn, *Hoyŏlja Chosŏn ŭl sŭpkyŏkhada: mom kwa ŭihak ŭi Hanguksa* [Cholera invades Chosŏn: History of the body and medicine in Korea] (Seoul: Yŏksa pip'yŏngsa, 2004). In English, see Donald Baker, "Oriental Medicine in Korea," in *Medicine Across Cultures: History and Practice of Medicine in Non-Western Cultures*, ed. H. Selin, 133–153 (Dordrecht, The Netherlands: Kluwer Academic Publishers, 2003); and Soyoung Suh, *Naming the Local: Medicine, Language, and Identity in Korea since the Fifteenth Century* (Cambridge, MA: Harvard University Asia Center, 2017).

12. Kim Ho, "18 segi huban kŏgyŏng sajok ŭi wisaeng kwa ŭiryo" [Health and medicine of capital-based elite families during the late eighteenth century], *Sŏul hak yŏngu* 11 (1998): 113–144.

13. Sin Tongwŏn, "Pyŏngang soegaro ingnŭn sŏng, pyŏng, chugŏm ŭi munhwasa" [Reading *Pyŏn'gang soegaro*, a cultural history of sexuality, disease, and death], *Yŏksa pip'yŏng* 67 (2004): 307–332. Moxibustion and acupuncture were practiced both at elite medical institutions and among the general populace. At the popular level, they might or might not be guided by the Sino-classical medical canon.

14. Yi Kkonme, "Hanguk ŭi udubŏp to'ip kwa silsi e kwanhan yŏngu: 1876 nyŏn esŏ 1910 nyŏn kkajirŭl chungsimŭro" [A study of the entrance and assimilation of cowpox vaccination in Korea, with a focus on the years between 1876 and 1910] (M.A. Thesis, Seoul National University, 1992). Human variolation technique was not as widespread as it was in Tokugawa Japan or China. In Chosŏn, it was often conducted by female healers who might or might not deploy shamanic explanations and practices in variolation. This accounts in part for some of the resistance and accommodations that took place with the introduction of vaccination in late Chosŏn.

15. One example is Yi Mungŏn (1494–1567) who penned *Yangarok* [Records of raising a child], a diary that recorded the education and health care he provided his grandson, his only surviving male descendant. In *Yangarok* there are references to his consulting fortune-tellers and following folk customs such as burial of the placenta. Yi Mungŏn, *Yangarok*, trans. Yi Sangju (Seoul: T'aehaksa, 1997).

16. Treaties with other states such as the United States (1882), Great Britain (1883), Germany (1883), Italy (1883), Russia (1884), France (1886), and Austria-Hungary (1889) soon followed. Before the general acceptance of the germ theory of contagion, application of antisepsis surgical methods, and use of mass-produced antibiotics, medical theories and therapeutics in Europe were no more or less effective than those in China. Rather, Rogaski suggests that any "divergence" and superiority Europe had lay in its better control of contagious disease due more to organization and administration than medical diagnosis and therapeutics. Ruth Rogaski, *Hygienic Modernity: Meaning of Health and Disease in Treaty-Port China* (Berkeley and Los Angeles: University of California Press, 2004).

17. Rogaski, *Hygienic Modernity*, 286.

18. Sin Tongwŏn details early discussions of Western modes of public sanitation in Korea in *Hanguk kŭndae pogŏn ŭiryosa* [History of health and medicine in modern Korea] (Seoul: Hanul Academy, 1997).

19. These activities were overseen by the T'ongni Amun ("Office for State Affairs," originally T'ongni Kimu Amun), the state organ formed to manage new responsibilities related to foreign affairs after Korea's entry in the Open Port period and modeled on the Chinese foreign office, the Tsungli Yamen. I indicate elsewhere that the fact that foreign offices initially managed medical and public health–related administration attests to the link made between health and state-building efforts in an

international context of competition and imperialism. Sonja Kim, "The Search for Health: Translating *Wisaeng* and Medicine During the Taehan Empire," in *Reform and Modernity in the Taehan Empire*, ed. Kim Dong-no, John B. Duncan, and Kim Do-hyung, 299–341 (Seoul: Jimoondang, 2006).

20. Chejungwŏn (literally, the "House of Succoring the People" and referred to as "His Majesty's Hospital" in mission reports) was originally named Kwanghyewŏn ("House of Extended Benevolence"). The Chosŏn court relinquished oversight of the hospital to missionaries in 1894. Chejungwŏn is the predecessor of today's Severance Hospital, affiliated with Yonsei University College of Medicine, a premier institution of medical education and care today in South Korea.

21. Andre Schmid calls the intellectual and physical process of rejecting, removing, or revising Sino-classical paradigms and institutions from their previous place of prominence the project of "decentering China." Andre Schmid, *Korea Between Empires, 1895–1919* (New York: Columbia University Press, 2002). The popular rebellion of 1894 that served as the pretext for the Sino-Japanese War grew from a local grievance over taxation to a mass movement that exhibited anti-foreign sentiments and demanded serious restructuring of local administration as well as social leveling. Some of the organizational networks and leadership of the Tonghak religion were involved in peasant mobilizations at this time, and thus these rebellions are commonly referred to today as the Tonghak Rebellion, or the Peasant War or Peasant Uprising of 1894. Sin Tongwŏn argues that the more aggressive application of new techniques from the West in the realm of health and medicine moved beyond the "Eastern Way, Western Techniques" to the "Old Foundation, New Participation" (*Kubon sinch'am*) framework adopted by the Taehan state.

22. For more on the politics of this period in the English language, see Kim et al., eds., *Reform and Modernity in the Taehan Empire*, and Kyung Moon Hwang, *Rationalizing Korea: The Rise of the Modern State, 1894–1945* (Oakland: University of California Press, 2016).

23. For an overview of public health and medical administration of this period in general, see Sin Tongwŏn, *Hanguk kŭndae pogŏn ŭiryosa*, and Pak Yunjae, *Hanguk kŭndae ŭihak ŭi kiwŏn* [The origin of the Korean modern medical system] (Seoul: Hyean, 2005). In English, see Todd Henry, "Sanitizing Empire: Articulations of Korean Otherness and the Construction of Early Colonial Seoul, 1905–1919," *Journal of Asian Studies* 64, no. 3 (2005): 639–675; Kyung Moon Hwang, *Rationalizing Korea*; Sonja Kim, "Search for Health"; and So Young Suh, "Korean Medicine

between the Local and the Universal: 1600–1945" (PhD diss., University of California, Los Angeles, 2006).

24. Sin Tongwŏn, *Hanguk kŭndae pogŏn ŭiryosa*, 198.

25. Pak Yunjae, "Taehan chegukki chongdu ŭi yangŏngso ŭi sŏllip kwa hwaltong" [Establishment of the training school for vaccinators and their activities during the Taehan Empire]," *Chŏngsin munhwa yŏngu* 32, no. 4 (2009): 29–54.

26. This hospital was originally called Hospital of the Interior before changing its name to Posiwŏn and immediately again to Kwangjewŏn. Operating as a relief hospital for the destitute, Kwangjewŏn resembled former welfare organs of the Chosŏn period based on the logic of extending the monarch's benevolence to his subjects. The newspaper *Hwangsŏng sinmun* indicated that physicians of both Western and Korean traditions were dispatched to treat sick prisoners. *Hwangsŏng sinmun*, March 2, 1899.

27. So Young Suh, "Korean Medicine between the Local and the Universal: 1600–1945," 103.

28. Pak Yunjae, "1876–1904 nyŏn Ilbon kwannip pyŏngwŏn ŭi sŏllip kwa hwaltong e kwanhan yŏngu" [A study on the establishment and activity of Japanese government hospitals in Korea, 1876–1904], *Yŏksa wa hyŏnsil* 42 (2001): 179–206.

29. I am using Ming-Cheng M. Lo's translation for Dōjinkai. Ming-Cheng M. Lo, *Doctors within Borders: Profession, Ethnicity, and Modernity in Colonial Taiwan* (Berkeley and Los Angeles: University of California Press, 2002), 153. The Dōjinkai in Korea received funding even from the Korean Taehan government. Pak Yunjae describes their activities in Korea in *Hanguk kŭndae ŭihak ŭi kiwŏn*, 148–163.

30. These public hospitals were initially called charity hospitals (*chahye ŭiwŏn*) and served the populace in outlying regions of the country. However, in an effort to save funds after the Kantō earthquake in 1923, the GGK changed the name to provincial hospitals (*torip ŭiwŏn*), removing their charitable function and shifting the financial burden to the public hospitals. Pak Yunjae, *Hanguk kŭndae ŭihak ŭi kiwŏn*, 266. When speaking of these public hospitals in general terms covering both before and after the name change, they will be designated as charity-provincial. When speaking of them at a specific historical moment, they will be identified by the name they used at that time.

31. The name Severance comes from the American Louis H. Severance, whose generous donation gave the hospital a new building and a firm foundation on which to grow.

32. Two examples of mission publications related to health are A.M. Sharrocks, *T'aemo wisaeng* [The hygiene of parturition] (Seoul: Methodist Publishing House, 1905) and J. H. Wells, *Wisaeng* [Introduction to hygiene], 2nd ed. (Seoul: Korean Religious Tract Society, 1907).

33. The public physician system in colonial Korea was apparently modeled on the successful public physician system in colonial Taiwan. Pak Yunjae, *Hanguk kŭndae ŭihak ŭi kiwŏn*, 267–274.

34. Ibid., 195–197.

35. As later chapters will attest, older practices of medicine associated with a Sino-classical tradition did not completely disappear but they did lose their place of prominence. These practices became reorganized under a new label "Korean medicine," then called *hanbang*, and often described as leading to the *hanŭi* practices of today under the current dual medical system practiced by the South Korean state. Nevertheless, the Japanese state aimed to implement what Sabine Frühstück identifies as a modern health regime of public health and medical services to build healthier bodies to serve in the military, work in expanding industries, and produce a larger population, elements of which were applied in its colonies. Sabine Frühstück, *Colonizing Sex: Sexology and Social Control in Modern Japan* (Berkeley and Los Angeles: University of California Press, 2003).

36. Ko Misuk argues that contrary to assumptions of Chosŏn society as prudish, at the turn of the twentieth century, women's sexuality was not so much repressed as it was dominated by their biological sexual function. *Hanguk kŭndaesŏng, kŭ kiwŏn ŭl ch'ajasŏ: minjok, seksyu'ŏllit'i, pyŏngnihak* [Finding the origin of Korea's modernity: Race, sexuality, pathology] (Seoul: Ch'ek sesang, 2001), 94.

37. Women deploying their authority as mothers played active roles in caretaking professions such as social work and district nursing, as well as in lobbying activities to promote the improvement of maternal health and infant care. Seth Koven and Sonya Michel, "Womanly Duties: Maternalist Politics and the Origins of the Welfare States in France, Germany, Great Britain, and the United States, 1880–1920," *American Historical Review* 95, no. 4 (1990): 1079.

38. I would like to thank Ruth Barraclough at the Australian National University who made this observation to me.

39. This definition of reproductive politics comes from Rickie Solinger, *Reproductive Politics: What Everyone Needs to Know* (New York: Oxford University Press, 2013). This monograph does not address reproductive politics comprehensively in terms of contraceptive or abortion rights, but more in terms of how the importance attached to female reproduction

by the state and medical field (care providers and researchers) shaped the ways women experienced transformations in medicine and public health.

40. Kim Hyegyŏng, *Singminjiha kŭndae kajok ŭi hyŏngsŏng chendŏ* [The formation of the modern family and gender during the colonial period] (Seoul: Ch'angbi Publications, 2006).

CHAPTER 1: SANITIZING WOMEN AND THE DOMESTIC SCIENCES

1. The two main powers that emerged in Korean affairs after the Sino-Japanese War were Japan and Russia, particularly as King Kojong made a dramatic escape from his palace to the Russian legation after the Japanese-masterminded assassination of his queen in 1896. Even after Kojong returned to his palace and declared himself emperor of the Taehan Empire in 1897, the constant jockeying at court among foreign delegates for favorable concessions was seen as signaling the weakness and lack of independent sovereignty of the state.

2. "Civilization and Enlightenment" (J. *bunmei kaika*) advocates promoted an aggressive form of modernization through active study and rapid appropriation of Western ideas and technologies modeled on Meiji Japan. A more moderate agenda, "Maintain Old Foundations, Add the New," expanded the self-strengthening framework of "Eastern Way, Western Techniques" to include selective adoption of new ideas and systems such as military technologies and bureaucratic institutions while preserving the intention to bolster the monarchical order. Scholars regard this as the source of guidelines adopted by Kojong and the Taehan state.

3. Martina Deuchler, *Confucian Transformation of Korea: A Study of Society and Ideology* (Cambridge, MA: Council on East Asian Studies and Harvard University Press, 1992).

4. Yu Kilchun (1856–1914) is considered one of the more radical and visionary reformers of late nineteenth-century Korea. His classical training, elite *yangban* status, and official appointment enabled him to study in Japan at Keio University and the United States at the Governor Dummer Academy (a private secondary school in Massachusetts), as well as to participate in fact-finding missions abroad. On his return to Korea in the aftermath of the 1884 Kapsin coup he was placed under house arrest, although he was abroad at the time of the failed coup attempt and was not directly linked to its planning. It was during this time that he recorded

his observations of social, political, and cultural practices in Korea in comparison with the West in a format similar to the works of Fukuzawa Yukichi, with whom he had studied in Japan. Although *Sŏyu kyŏnmun* was not published until 1894, Yu's ideas are consistent with the progressive thinkers of his time generally labeled as affiliated with "Enlightenment" (*kaehwa*) thinking. The edition of *Sŏyu kyŏnmun* cited here is Yu Kilchun, *Sŏyu kyŏnmun*, trans. Hŏ Kyŏngjin (Seoul: Sŏhae munjip, 2004). English translations are from Yu Kilchun, "Observations on a Journey to the West," ed. John B. Duncan, trans. Hanmee Na Kim et al. (unpublished manuscript, January 25, 2017), Microsoft Word file.

5. For more on female education during the Chosŏn dynasty, see Song Insu, *Hanguk yŏsŏng kyoyuksa* [History of Korean women's education] (Seoul: Yonsei University Press, 1977); John Duncan, "The *Naehun* and the Politics of Gender in Fifteenth-Century Korea," in *Creating Women of Korea: The Fifteenth through the Twentieth Centuries*, ed. Young-Key Kim-Renaud (Armonk, NY, and London: M. E. Sharpe, 2004), 26–57; and Martina Deuchler, "Propagating Female Virtues in Chosŏn Korea," in *Women and Confucian Cultures in Premodern China, Korea, and Japan*, ed. Dorothy Ko, Ja-Hyun Haboush, and Joan Piggott (Berkeley, Los Angeles, and London: University of California Press, 2003), 142–169.

6. According to Se-mi Oh, petitions and circular letters began to shift in this period from private or closed circuits of communication to public discussion through the medium of newspapers, often being reprinted in multiple publications at roughly the same time. The Ch'anyanghoe's petition referred here followed Chosŏn forms of communication between a petitioner and the king but became publicly known as it was published in the *Independent*, *Daily News*, and *Imperial Post* on October 13, 1898. Se-mi Oh, "Letters to the Editor: Women, Newspapers, and the Public Sphere in Turn-of-the Century Korea," in *Epistolary Letters: Letters in the Communicative Space of the Chosŏn, 1392–1910*, ed. Ja-Hyun Kim Haboush (New York: Columbia University Press, 2009), 162–167.

7. Kim-ssi of Yanghyŏndang established Chŏngsŏn Girls' School in Seoul in 1897 using private funds. Due to financial difficulties, it closed in 1903. Song Insu, *Hanguk yŏsŏng kyoyuksa*, 246. Ewha Girls' School (*Ewha haktang*), predecessor to Korea's premier women's college Ewha Womans University, was established in 1886 by Methodist missionary Mary F. Scranton. Over the years, Ewha developed a middle-high school, kindergarten teacher training school, and college. The spelling of the university used is its official English name as listed on its website. https://www.ewha.ac.kr/mbs/ewhaen/.

8. Translated selections used here are from Se-mi Oh, "Letters to the Editor," 163.

9. Hansŏng Girls' High School was later taken over by the GGK, renamed Keijō Girls' Higher Common School (*Kyŏngsŏng yŏja kodŭng pot'ong hakkyo*, discussed later in the chapter) and the predecessor of Kyŏnggi Girls' High School, considered the premier girls' high school in post-1945 South Korea. *Kyŏnggi yŏgo 100 nyŏnsa* [100 years of Kyŏnggi Girls' High School] (Seoul: Kyŏngunhoe, 2009).

10. Chosŏn had a rigid hierarchical social order with *yangban*, consisting of the *sadaebu* or scholar-official literati families at the top, followed by secondary status groups such as military and regional officials as well as technician-bureaucrat *chungin*, commoners, and the lowest *ch'ŏnmin* status that included slaves and those in base or mean occupations such as butchers, tanners, and female entertainers. For more on Chosŏn's social status system, see Kyung Moon Hwang, *Beyond Birth: Social Status in the Emergence of Modern Korea* (Cambridge, MA: Harvard University Asia Center, 2004).

11. Some of these publications include the 1518 vernacular translation of *Elementary Learning* (Ch. *Xiaoxue*; K. *Sohak*), a primer of moral lessons by Zhu Xi, and illustrated texts of the three cardinal human relationships (between ruler and subject, parent and child, husband and wife) such as the *Illustrated Guide to the Three Bonds* (*Samgang haengsilto*, 1432), which was reprinted on several occasions, modifications in later editions reflecting social changes. See Martina Deuchler, "Propagating Female Virtues in Chosŏn Korea." For more discussion of neo-Confucian social engineering during the Chosŏn dynasty, see Martina Deuchler, *The Confucian Transformation of Korea*. Deuchler argues that despite legislation passed in the early years of the dynasty, such engineering took a few centuries to transform Chosŏn's kinship and social system.

12. Deuchler asserts that, while not immediate, over the centuries "the new state ideology altered [women's] social standing, their place within family and kin group, and their relations to the nondomestic outside world." Martina Deuchler, "Propagating Female Virtues in Chosŏn Korea," 143.

13. A son of a secondary wife or remarried widow, for example, did not qualify to sit for the civil service examination. Official recognition of a daughter-in-law's exemplary display of female chastity, reflected most extremely in suicide, could bring material and symbolic gains to her husband's family.

14. The Chosŏn legal code delineated various punitive measures for female transgressions such as corporal punishment for adultery. The

disqualification of her sons from the civil service examination upon her remarriage could also be considered punitive. On the other hand, the Chosŏn legal framework allowed for and encouraged women to advocate for their interests in the legal system, albeit on behalf of the lineage. See Jisoo M. Kim, *Emotions of Justice: Gender, Status, and Legal Performance in Chosŏn Korea* (Seattle: University of Washington Press, 2016).

15. Some official publications include the *Illustrated Guide to the Three Bonds*, translations of Chinese didactic texts such as *Biographies of Exemplary Women* (Ch. *Lienü zhuan*; K. *Yŏllyŏ chŏn*), the *Precepts for Women* (Ch. *Nüjie*; K. *Yŏgye*), and the *Rules for Women* (Ch. *Nüze*; K. *Yŏch'ik*). Other translations include those ordered by King Yŏngjo in the eighteenth century of the *Four Books for Women* (Ch. *Nü sishu*; K. *Yŏ sasŏ ŏnhae*). Martina Deuchler, "Propagating Female Virtues." Conscientious parents instructed their daughters from a young age, enforcing reading (facilitated by vernacular editions) and/or recitation (a popular pedagogical method in Chosŏn to memorize Confucian classics). According to Michael J. Pettid, private texts for elite women fell broadly into three categories: texts which covered a woman's life from childhood, texts which oriented her toward life after marriage, and guides or advice books written by her father. While they maintained the didactic flavor of official publications, they also carried more practical advice, particularly for a woman's future roles in her husband's household. Michael J. Pettid, "Confucian Educational Works for Upper Status Women in Chosŏn," in *Women and Confucianism in Chosŏn Korea*, ed. Michael J. Pettid and Youngmin Kim (Albany: State University of New York Press, 2011), 49–70.

16. Description of these board games can be found in Michael J. Pettid, "Confucian Educational Works for Upper Status Women in Chosŏn." Some precepts that emerge in *naebang* or *kyubang kasa* include how to serve one's parents-in-law, prepare ancestral offerings, manage household servants and the budget. The *naebang kasa "Kyonyŏ ka"* in particular was composed by a father for his youngest daughter upon her marriage. Sonja Häußler, "Kyubang Kasa: Women's Writings from the Late Chosŏn," in *Creative Women of Korea*, 142–162.

17. Adoption (by placing the name of the adopted heir on the family registry and genealogy) of male relatives in the next generation, usually a nephew (not sons conceived with women other than the primary wife, sons-in-law as practiced in Japan, or other men), became the practice among *sadaebu* families in the Chosŏn period to ensure legitimate succession when a biological male heir was unavailable. Martina Deuchler, *The Confucian Transformation of Korea.* From personal communications, I know

that this form of "adoption" of male relatives, while uncommon, continued in the twentieth century among older generations.

18. My analysis of *Kyuhap ch'ongsŏ* comes from a reading of its reprint, Pinghŏgak Yi ssi, *Kyuhap ch'ongsŏ*, trans. Yi Minsu (Seoul: Kirinwŏn, 1988).

19. This section in *Kyuhap ch'ongsŏ* was titled "*T'aegyo*" ("fetal education" or "education in the womb"), which remains today as an umbrella term that indicates a broad range of cultural practices in the consumer market in South Korea related to prenatal care and the education of the unborn child. The *Tongŭi pogam* is credited to the famed court physician Hŏ Chun and is considered a masterly synthesis of Chinese classical medical texts and Korean indigenous medical knowledge. While it was only one of several texts referenced by physicians, the *Tongŭi pogam* has become understood as the quintessential text in nativist articulations of a Korean medical tradition, distinct from Chinese medicine. It continues today as a reference in the Korean Medicine (*hanŭi*) field. Sin Tongwŏn, Kim Namil, and Yŏ Insŏk, *Han kwŏnŭro ingnŭn* Tongŭi pogam [Reading the *Tongŭi pogam* in one volume] (Seoul: Tŭllyŏk, 1999).

20. *T'aegyo singi* was written in 1800 by Madam Yi of Sajudang (1739–1821) and circulated privately. Amid the publication of new literature for use in female education, it was published serially for public consumption in 1908 in the journal of the academic society Kiho Hŭnghakhoe.

21. An T'aeyun, *Singmin chŏngch'i wa mosŏng: ch'ongdongwŏn ch'eje wa mosŏng ŭi hyŏnsil* [The politics of motherhood in colonial Korea] (P'aju, South Korea: Hanguk haksul chŏngbo, 2006), 50.

22. Writing with the right hand would enable men to write properly with brush and ink, a paramount activity of the Confucian scholar-gentleman. Analysis of *Naehun* is based on the translated version in Chohŏn wanghu Han ssi and Song Siyŏl, *Sinwanyŏk Naehun, Kyenyŏsŏ*, trans. Kim Chonggwŏn (Seoul: Myŏngmundang, 1987). For more on the text *Naehun*, see John Duncan, "The *Naehun* and Politics of Gender in Fifteenth-Century Korea."

23. *Chŭngbo sannim kyŏngje* was an expanded edition of Hong Mansŏn's agrarian manual *Sannim kyŏngje*, compiled by Ryu Chungnim, a palace physician. Two of its sixteen chapters were devoted to *kajŏng*. While the author of the independent volume also titled *Kajŏng* is unknown, its content is similar to that of the *Kajŏng* section in *Chŭngbo sannim kyŏngje*, suggesting male authorship. Agrarian manuals in general were not considered part of the curriculum for aspiring civil service exam candidates but part of the larger erudition expected of the landed elite

and in this way can be likened to other Chosŏn period medical texts or household manuals. Yi Sugin, "'Kajŏng' (家政) ŭl t'onghae pon 18 segi ŭi saenghwal segye" [Eighteenth-century everyday life as seen through *Kajŏng*], *Hanguk munhwa* 51 (2010): 65–88.

24. Some elite women were well educated and literate in classical Chinese but this was not very common.

25. Jisoo M. Kim, "From Jealousy to Violence: Marriage, Family, and Confucian Patriarchy in Fifteenth Century Korea," *Acta Koreana* 20, no. 1 (2017): 91–110.

26. Sin Yongha, "Uri nara ch'oech'o ŭi kŭndae hakkyo sŏllip e taehayŏ" [On the establishment of the first modern school in Korea], *Hanguksa yŏngu* 10, no. 9 (1974): 191–204. For an overview of Korean education in this period, see *Hanguk kŭndae hakkyo kyoyuk 100 nyŏnsa yŏngu* [One hundred years of the history of education in Korean modern schools], vol. 1 (Seoul: Hanguk kyoyuk kaebarwŏn, 1994); Klaus Dittrich, "The Beginnings of Modern Education in Korea, 1883–1910," *Paedagogica Histories* 50, no. 3 (2014): 265–284; and Leighanne Kimberly Yuh, "Education, the Struggle for Power, and Identity Formation in Korea, 1876–1910" (PhD diss., University of California, Los Angeles, 2008).

27. These first government schools, however, did not last more than a decade. Leighanne Kimberly Yuh, "Guns, Farms, and Foreign Languages: The Introduction of Western Learning and the First Government Schools in Late Nineteenth-Century Korea," *Paedagogica Historica* 52, no. 6 (2016): 580–595.

28. While Korean historiography often credits missionaries with contributing significantly to the modernization of Korea, particularly in the areas of education, medicine, and the status of women, the evangelizing agenda of mission schools constrained the curriculum and operation of the schools which were foremost to be the means to lead Koreans to Christ. Leighanne Yuh points out that there was a "strict mission board policy . . . to set up a few schools with high standards 'for Christian work'" aimed to ameliorate Korean distrust of missionaries and fulfill God's work, with little intention of establishing modern mass education. "Education, the Struggle for Power," 107. Hyaeweol Choi analyzes how Christian imperatives shaped girls' mission schools, which some of its students critiqued. Hyaeweol Choi, *Gender and Mission Encounters: New Women, Old Ways* (Berkeley: University of California Press, 2009).

29. Other contested terms include modernization, democracy, rights, and equality, among others.

30. Kyung Moon Hwang, *Rationalizing Korea*, 168–194. Hwang does not suggest that the public school system was a completed project in citizenship education but rather an ongoing process in the *making* of citizens, however defined by the state in power at the time. He also observes that under the Japanese colonial administration, *kungmin* was de-coupled from conceptualizations of the ethnic nation, or *minjok*.

31. The original text of the 1895 Educational Edict may be found digitally on the website Korean history net (http://contents.history.go.kr/), which is managed by the National Institute of Korean History (*Kuksa p'yŏnch'an wiwŏnhoe*), a major repository of archival sources and promoter of academic research in Korean history. The decree was originally published in the official gazette *Kwanbo* in 1895, 2nd lunar month, 2nd day. English translation of the title *Kyoyuk ipkuk chosŏ* comes from Leighanne Yuh, "Education, the Struggle for Power," 156. Translations and analysis of the decree itself are my own.

32. Kim Minjae, "Kŭndae susin kyogwasŏ t'amsaek ŭl t'onghan chŏnt'ong kyoyuk kwa hyŏndae todŏkkwa kyoyuk ŭi yŏngyŏl" [Looking at traditional education and contemporary ethics education through *susin* textbooks], in *Kŭndae hakpu p'yŏnch'an susinsŏ* [*Susin* textbooks published by the modern board of education], ed. Pak Pyŏnggi and Kim Minjae (Seoul: Somyŏng, 2012), 212–222.

33. South Korean public elementary schools as of 2017 still offer an ethics course called *Todŏk*. There is a long-standing historiographical debate over whether Korea's modernizing transformation involved ruptures, continuities, or a combination of both; and the role of the Japanese imperial system in the transition from the Chosŏn period to post-1945 Korean society. Scholars' interpretations vary, focusing on diverse sectors including commerce, industry, agriculture, communications, transportation, gender relations and family structure, education, law, mass media, leisure and popular culture, professionalization, public health and medicine, religion, and social organization, to name a few. Nevertheless, there is a general consensus that moral values associated with or directly claiming Confucian origins have proved useful in mobilizing and organizing Koreans since the nineteenth century. This chapter focuses on the moral imperatives in the realms of education and gender.

34. Leighanne Kimberly Yuh, "Moral Education, Modernization Imperatives, and the People's Elementary Reader (1895): Accommodation in the Early History of Modern Education in Korea," *Acta Koreana* 18, no. 2 (2015): 327–355.

35. Mary F. Scranton, the founder of Ewha Girls' School, stated that mission education was to make "Koreans better Koreans" by working toward a "perfect Korea through Christ and his teachings." As cited in Theodore Jun Yoo, *Politics of Gender in Colonial Korea: Education, Labor, and Health, 1910–1945* (Berkeley and Los Angeles: University of California Press, 2008), 48.

36. The protectorate aroused much protest, including the armed resistance of the Righteous Armies (*ŭibyŏng*) and political suicides of high-profile figures such as Min Yŏnghwan. It also created a sense of betrayal among Koreans, especially those who had previously looked to Japan as a model and adopted a pan-Asianist orientation in pursuing a modernizing agenda. Japan's increasing interventions in Korean affairs included jurisdiction in handling Korea's diplomatic affairs, the forced dethroning of Kojong in 1907, disarmament of the Korean militia, tightening the censorship of print media, and gradually assuming administration of domestic affairs. The time from 1905–1910 is often referred to as a period of "Patriotic Enlightenment," as concerned Koreans engaged in a flurry of cultural and educational activities. See Andre Schmid, *Korea Between Empires*.

37. Government General of Chosen, *Manual of Education in Chosen* (1920), reprinted in *Singminji Chosŏn kyoyuk chŏngch'aek saryo chipsŏng* [Sources on educational policy in colonial Korea], vol. 2 (Seoul: Taehaksŏwon, 1990).

38. The professional (*chŏnmun*; J. *senmon*) level of education referred to advanced specialized training such as medicine. Schools designated as professional schools will be translated as college. Graduation from an accredited high school (not part of the common [*pot'ong*] curriculum), preparatory course, or passing an examination were often required for entrance into a professional school. The curriculum at higher common schools (*kodŭng pot'ong*) offered to Koreans after primary school is likened to middle school in Japan.

39. "Instructions Concerning the Enforcement of the Chosen Educational Ordinance" (1911), in *Manual of Education in Chosen*, 12.

40. Articles 4 and 8 respectively of the 1911 Educational Ordinance, *Manual on Education of* Chosen, 1–2. Until revision of the 1911 Educational Ordinance in 1922, the GGK offered only four years of schooling at primary grade levels. Even after extending the primary school curriculum to six years, the GGK did not offer high school education beyond the higher common level besides vocational training to Korean students. Students who sought higher education at specialized schools to practice medicine

or teach school would often have to take additional preparatory courses to make up for their lack of high school level education.

41. After the 1922 revision of the Educational Ordinance, the maximum tuition for Japanese students was 50 sen whereas for Korean students, it was 1 yen (100 sen). Poverty was listed by Koreans as a major reason why they did not send their children to public schools. Kim Puja, *Hakkyo pak ŭi Chosŏn yŏsŏngtŭl* [Korean women outside of school], trans. Cho Kyŏnghŭi and Kim Uja (Seoul: Ilchogak, 2005), 107.

42. For more on education in colonial Korea, see *Hanguk kŭndae hakkyo kyoyuk 100 nyŏnsa yŏngu* [One hundred years of the history of education in Korean modern schools], vol. 2 (Seoul: Hanguk kyoyuk kaebarwŏn, 1997); Kang Myŏngsuk, *Sarip hakkyo ŭi kiwŏn: Ilche ch'ogi hakkyo sŏllip kwa chiyŏk sahoe* [Origins of private schools: Establishment of schools and local society in early colonial Korea] (Seoul: Hagi sisŭp, 2015); O Sŏngch'ŏl, *Singminji ch'odŭng kyoyuk ŭi hyŏngsŏng* [Formation of elementary education in the colonial period] (Seoul: Kyoyuk kwahaksa, 2000); and O Sŏngch'ŏl, ed., *Singminji kyoyuk yongu ŭi tabyŏnhwa* [Diversification of studies on colonial period education] (P'aju, South Korea: Kyoyuk kwahaksa, 2011).

43. While the techniques and efficacy of assimilation practices in general to cultivate a self-regulating and managed population of subjects are beyond the scope of this book, the important point here is that prescribed roles and desired relationships between subjects and the state directed the design of curriculum and the operation of public schools in both the Taehan and colonial periods. The assimilationist character of colonial education remains a bitter feature of Korean public memory of the colonial period, particularly in narratives of the eradication of Korean culture, language, and national identity. For discussion on the Japanese imperialist agenda as reflected in GGK-published ethics textbooks, see Kim Sunjŏn et al., *Cheguk ŭi singminji susin: Chosŏn ch'ongdokpu p'yŏnch'an Susinsŏ yŏngu* [Colonial ethics in the empire: Study of ethics textbooks published by the GGK] (Seoul: JENC, 2009). For more on assimilation practices in general, see Mark E. Caprio, *Japanese Assimilation Policies in Colonial Korea, 1910–1945* (Seattle: University of Washington Press, 2009) and Todd Henry, *Assimilating Seoul: Japanese Rule and the Politics of Public Space in Colonial Korea, 1910–1945* (Berkeley: University of California Press, 2014).

44. Kim Sunjŏn and Cho Sŏngjin, "Ilcheha Chosŏn kyoyuk ŭi hyŏngsang kwa chanjae: tonghwa wa ch'abyŏl ŭl chungsimŭro" [Situation and vestiges of Korean education under Japanese imperialism: Assimilation

and discrimination], in *Cheguk ŭi singminji susin*, ed. Kim Sunjŏn, et al. (Seoul: JENC, 2009), 251–282. It is interesting to note that the name *kungmin hakkyo* to refer to primary schools was used in South Korea until recent times. As a decolonization gesture, the name of primary schools was changed to *ch'odŭng hakkyo* (elementary schools) in 1996.

45. GGK schools beyond the primary level, however, were sex-segregated for the most part.

46. Analysis of the textbooks discussed here and *Common School Morals Textbook* come from their reprint in Pak Pyŏnggi and Kim Minjae, trans., *Kŭndae hakpu p'yonch'an* Susinsŏ [Ethics textbooks published by the modern board of education] (Seoul: Somŏng ch'ulp'an, 2012).

47. Leighanne Kimberly Yuh, "Moral Education."

48. For example, both the protectorate period and GGK ethics textbooks open with the lesson "School." Other similar lessons include: caring for one's possessions, cleanliness and care of one's body, and lying as a vice. GGK ethics textbooks were reprinted (1913, 1922, 1928, 1939, and 1943) throughout the colonial period, usually in conjunction with major revisions to the Educational Ordinance. The GGK textbooks I used for analysis are from their reprint in Kim Sunjŏn, ed., *Chosŏn ch'ongdokpu ch'odŭng hakkyo susinso* [GGK's elementary school ethics textbooks], vols. 1–2 (Seoul: JENC, 2006).

49. The 1922 edition was published in the context of the 1922 revisions to the Educational Ordinance in the aftermath of the series of Korean nationalist-inspired demonstrations and protests collectively called the March 1st (3.1) movement of 1919.

50. Cited in Se-mi Oh, "Letters to the Editor," 63.

51. "Nyŏ hakkyo ron," *Tongnip sinmun*, May 26, 1899. The *Tongnip sinmun* (The Independent, 1896–1899), the first Korean newspaper written completely in the Korean phonetic script (and with an English edition) was started by Sŏ Chaep'il (Philip Jaisohn) who had spent a decade in exile studying in the United States in the aftermath of the 1884 Kapsin coup in which he was a participant. His Christian background and proclivity for American models of civic governance are reflected in the activities he helped organize and in editorials. The English edition of the paper will be referenced as *The Independent*, whereas the Korean edition will be referenced by its Korean title.

52. *Tongnip sinmun*, February 10, 1898, translation by Ji-Eun Lee, *Women Pre-Scripted: Forging Modern Roles through Korean Print* (Honolulu: University of Hawai'i Press, 2015), 47.

53. Hyaeweol Choi, "The Missionary Home as a Pulpit: Domestic Paradoxes in Early Twentieth-Century Korea," in *Divine Domesticities: Christian Paradoxes in Asia and the Pacific*, ed. Margaret Jolly and Hyaeweol Choi (Canberra: Australian National University Press, 2014), 29–55.

54. An argument to cultivate compatible wives is cited in Theodore Jun Yoo, *Politics of Gender in Colonial Korea*, 55. The logic advocating education to cultivate wives fit for the modern man is repeated in later 1920s and 1930s discourses on female students and the New Woman. Kim Sujin, *Sin yŏsŏng, kŭndae ŭi kwa'ing: singminji Chosŏn ŭi sin yŏsŏng tamnon kwa chendŏ chŏngch'i, 1920–1934* [Excess of the modern: The new woman in colonial Korea] (Seoul: Somyŏng ch'ulp'an, 2009).

55. *Tongnip sinmun*, May 12, 1896, translation by Ji-Eun Lee, *Women Pre-Scripted*, 47.

56. Ji-Eun Lee, *Women Pre-Scripted*, 45.

57. Jordan Sand, *House and Home in Modern Japan: Architecture, Domestic Space, and Bourgeois Culture, 1880–1930* (Cambridge, MA: Harvard University Press, 2004), 25–26.

58. Ibid., 21.

59. This conclusion is based on reading various treatises on *kajŏng kyoyuk* in early textbooks and bulletins from academic societies. For example, the female primer *Yŏja tokpon* (1908) declared that *kajŏng kyoyuk* led citizens (*kungmin*) to the right path of learning.

60. "Kajŏng kyoyuk ŭi t'ŭkjil" [Features of home education], *Sŏbuk hakhoe wŏlbo* 13 (1909): 3–6.

61. As reprinted in Hŏ Chaeyŏng et al., ed. and trans., *Kŭndae susin kyogwasŏ* [Modern moral textbooks] (Seoul: Somyŏng ch'ulp'an, 2011), 155. While not explicitly stated, the children here are likely two sons and a daughter, based on their hairstyles in the illustration.

62. The Chinese characters for Wise Mother, Good Wife in Korea were the same as Japan's Good Wife, Wise Mother but in reverse order. Scholars disagree on whether the order marked disparity between Korean and Japanese gender ideologies, prioritization of the role of the wife or the mother, facility of language, or nothing at all.

63. See Sharon Nolte and Sally Ann Hastings, "The Meiji State's Policy Toward Women, 1890–1910," in *Recreating Japanese Women, 1600–1945*, ed. Gail Lee Bernstein (Berkeley: University of California Press, 1991), 151–174, and Koyama Shizuko, *Ryōsai Kenbo: The Educational Ideal of "Good Wife, Wise Mother" in Modern Japan*, trans. Stephen Filler (Leiden: Brill, 2013).

64. Linda L. Johnson, "Meiji Women's Educators as Public Intellectuals: Shimoda Utako and Tsuda Umeko," *U.S.-Japan Women's Journal* 44 (2014): 73.

65. Foreign missionaries sought to build "Christian homes" with modern housekeeping, situating a woman as the "'moral arbiter' in nurturing children and fostering a loving conjugal relationship" based in part on ideals of Victorian womanhood. Hyaeweol Choi, "'Wise Mother, Good Wife': A Transcultural Discursive Construct in Modern Korea," *The Journal of Korean Studies* 14, no. 1 (2009): 11.

66. This accounts for the rationale in Chosŏn legal codes to assign heavier punishment for the same crime on those from higher social status groups. This also accounts for why legal stipulations against widow remarriage applied only to primary wives of *yangban* status by disqualifying their sons' eligibility to sit for the civil service examination. This did not mean, however, that socially prescribed values and behavior were exercised exclusively by the elite. Also, a mother-in-law may take more liberties and possess more authority than, for example, the youngest daughter-in-law of the youngest generation.

67. Hyaeweol Choi suggests that this was perhaps more prominent in Korea than in Japan on account of the large gap in educational opportunities between female students in Japan and Korea. Hyaeweol Choi, "Wise Mother, Good Wife," 9.

68. The *Ewha kajŏnghak 50 nyŏnsa* [Fifty-year history of home economics at Ewha] (Seoul: Ihwa yŏja taehak kajŏng taehak, 1979) records that courses offered to the first students at Ewha Girls' School were in English, the Bible, reading and writing the vernacular (*ŏnmun*), and composition. Physiology (*saengnihak*) was added in 1889 before female arts such as opera, organ (1891), and academic subjects such as classical Chinese, arithmetic, geography, history, and science (1892). See page 34. Ewha's first classes in household manual arts were in 1896. *Kajŏng kwahak taehak 70 nyŏnsa* [Seventy-year history of domestic science college] (Seoul: Ingan saenghwal hwangyŏng yŏnguso, 1999).

69. Sand, *House and Home in Modern Japan*, 58.

70. This is similar to the case of *wisaeng*, which was often conflated with the more familiar lexicon of health-preservation techniques known as *yangsaeng* (J. *yōshō*; Ch. *yangsheng*). See Pak Yunjae, "Yangsaengesŏ wisaengŭro, kaehwap'a ŭi ŭihangnon kwa kŭndae kukka kŏnsŏl" [From yangsaeng to wisaeng, medical discourse of the Kaehwa group and construction of the modern state], *Sahoe wa yŏksa* [Society and history] 63 (2003): 30–50, and Sonja Kim, "Search for Health."

71. Song Insu, *Hanguk yŏsŏng kyoyuksa*, 238.

72. The Regulations are reprinted in Song Insu, *Hanguk yŏsŏng kyoyuksa*, 238–239. The *Tongnip sinmun* also discusses the content of the Regulations. "Nyo Hakkyo," *Tongnip sinmun*, May 26, 1899.

73. While educational decrees and regulations of 1895 do not necessarily indicate that educational reforms were male sex-specific, early activities in public schooling were geared toward the male student. The exclusion of females is reinforced by the fact that separate regulations, edicts, and schools were established for girls.

74. Leighanne Kimberly Yuh, "Education, the Struggle for Power," 165. The age maximum of fifteen years at girls' schools was likely due to the Korean custom of marrying daughters before their early twenties.

75. Hyŏn hailed from an illustrious family of translators of Chinese texts. Kim Kyŏngnam, "Kŭndae kyemonggi kajŏnghak yŏksul choryorŭl t'onghae pon chisik suyong yangsik" [Accommodation of knowledge as seen through the translated compilations on *kajŏnghak* in the modern enlightenment period], *Inmun kwahak yŏngu* [Studies in the humanities] 46 (2015): 5–28.

76. In the preface, Hyŏn did not provide a title of the Chinese work on which he based his translation but credited the illustrious Chinese educator and first chancellor of Beijing University Wu Rulun for the Chinese translation of Shimoda's text. Wu visited with Shimoda at the Peeresses' and her Practical Arts schools. Shimoda actively promoted the education of Chinese women, pursuing a Chinese translation of her textbook and accepting many students in her schools so that by 1907 one-third of her student population at the Practical Arts School were Chinese foreign students. I have not been able to confirm the title or translator for this Chinese text. On Shimoda Utako, see Paula Harrell, "The Meiji 'New Woman' and China," in *Late Qing China and Meiji Japan: Political and Cultural Aspects*, ed. Joshua A. Fogel (Norwalk, CT: EastBridge, 2004), 109–150, and Linda L. Johnson, "Meiji Women's Educators as Public Intellectuals."

77. According to Linda Johnson, based on her experiences abroad, teaching, and public speaking, Shimoda developed a female curriculum that combined "Western technical skills (domestic science, mathematics, and science) with instruction in traditional Japanese feminine virtues." Linda Johnson, "Meiji Women's Educators as Public Intellectuals," 74.

78. Lydia Liu, *Translingual Practice: Literature, National Culture, and Translated Modernity—China, 1900–1937* (Redwood City, CA: Stanford University Press, 1995).

79. Most of the scientific treatises published by academic societies at this time were translations based on Chinese texts. See Chŏn Migyŏng,

"1900–1910 nyŏndae kajŏng kyogwasŏ e kwanhan yŏngu: Hyŏn Kongnyŏm parhaeng *Hanmun kajŏnghak, Sinp'yŏn kajŏnghak, Sinjŏng kajŏnghak ŭl chungsimŭro*" [A study of home economics textbooks in the 1900–1910s: An analysis of *Hanmun kajŏnghak, Sinp'yŏn kajŏnghak,* and *Sinjŏng kajŏnghak* published by Hyŏn Kongnyŏm], *Hanguk kajŏngkwa kyoyukhak hoeji* [Journal of Korean Home Economics Education] 16, no. 3 (2004): 1–25; 17, no. 1 (2005): 136–137; and Pak Chongsŏk, "Kaehwagi kwahak kyoyukcha ŭi paegyŏng kwa yŏkhwal" [Background and role of science educators of the Kaehwa period], Hanguk kwahak kyoyukhak hoeji [Journal of Korean Science Education], 20, no. 3 (2000): 443–454.

80. Unfortunately, it was not common practice for translators to indicate the original source of their translations.

81. Chŏn Migyŏng provides information on the Chinese text and a table of contents for Shimoda's text in "1900–1910 nyŏndae kajŏng kyogwasŏ e kwanhan yŏngu." Analysis of Hyŏn's texts are based on my reading of the original texts archived at Ewha Womans University library.

82. Shimoda's text consisted of two volumes. Hyŏn's translations were only one volume.

83. Chang Chiyŏn, *Yŏja tokpon* (1908), ed. and trans., Mun Hyeyun (Kwangmyŏng, South Korea: Kyŏngjin, 2012). On presentations of womanhood in early female textbooks, see Pak Yongok, "1905–1910 nyŏn sŏgu kŭndae yŏsŏngsang e taehan ohae wa insik [Understanding of Western modern womanhood, 1905–1910]," *Hanguk yŏsŏng kŭndaehwa ŭi yŏksachŏk maengnak*, 297–339 (Seoul: Chisik sanŏpsa, 2001); Cho Kyŏngwŏn, "Taehan cheguk mal yŏhaksaeng kyogwasŏ e nat'anan yŏsŏng kyoyuk ron ŭi t'ŭksŏng kwa hangye [A content analysis of textbooks for female students in the end of the Taehan empire period]," *Kyoyuk kwahak yŏngu* [Research in education science] 30 (1999): 163–187; and Kim Ŏnsun, "Kaehwagi yŏsŏng kyoyuk e naejaechŏk yŏsŏnggwan [Perspectives of women on the education of women in the period of Enlightenment]," *P'eminijŭm yŏngu* [Feminism] 10, no. 2 (2010): 35–87.

84. No Pyŏnghŭi, *Yŏja sohak sushinsŏ*, reprinted in Hanguk munhŏn yŏnguso, ed. *Hanguk kaehwagi kyogwasŏ ch'ongsŏ* [Collection of textbooks from the *kaehwa* period] 10 (Seoul: Asea munhwasa, 1977), 535–614.

85. "Yŏja susin ch'ongnon [Outline of female ethics]," chapter 53 of *Yŏja sohak susinsŏ* (1977), 613.

86. Yi Ki, "Kajŏnghak sŏl," *Honam hakpo* 1 (1908), 30.

87. Todd Henry, *Assimilating Seoul* and "Sanitizing Empire." For example, the colonial government insisted on salubrious habits and everyday practices as befitting civilized people to guard the colony against contagions.

88. Government textbooks for physical education appear in the colonial period with *Ch'ejo* [Calisthenics]. According to the instructors' manual, *wisaeng* principles were to be taught alongside the exercises illustrated in the textbook. All figures demonstrating the exercises in the 1924 textbook are male. GGK, *(Sohakkyo pot'ong hakkyo) ch'ejo kyosuyong chŏn* [Calisthenics for elementary and common schools, instructor edition] (1924).

89. An Chonghwa, trans., *Ch'odŭng yulli kyogwasŏ* [Elementary ethics textbook] (1907), 1–2, reprinted in *Hanguk kaehwagi kyogwasŏ ch'ongsŏ* 10, 480–481.

90. Note that these are the three areas of education (physical, moral, and knowledge) articulated in Kojong's 1895 proclamations on education.

91. This is based on analysis of *susin* textbooks such as Pak Chŏngdong's *Ch'odŭng susin* [Elementary morals] (1909), reprinted in *Hanguk kaehwagi kyogwasŏ ch'ongsŏ* 9 (Seoul: Asea munhwasa, 1977), 81–158, and those produced by the GGK, *Ch'odŭng hakkyo susinsŏ* [Elementary morals textbook; J. *Shotō gakkō shūshinsho*] which underwent several revisions but continued to provide instructions on *wisaeng*.

92. An Chonghwa, trans., *Ch'odŭng saengni wisaenghak taeyo* [An elementary outline on physiology and hygiene] (Hansŏng (Seoul): Kwangdŏk sŏgwan, 1909).

93. For example, lessons 2 (laundry) and 7 (food), Grade 2 in the 1913 edition.

94. There were one or two examples of boys sweeping the yard.

95. For example, "Clean Bodies," Lesson 8, Grade 1 (1928); "Public Hygiene," Lesson 7, Grade 5 (1928).

96. Yi Ki, "Kajŏnghak sŏl," 30.

97. One example is Lesson 12 in the Grade 4 ethics common school textbook (1907). This lesson appears in GGK ethics textbooks as well. "Philanthropy," Lesson 16, Grade 4 (1922). These lessons present Nightingale as nursing with a heart of compassion and charity. Nightingale is also seen as a major inspiration for missionaries and Japanese in the field of nursing, especially for the latter in her contributions on the battlefield.

98. Pak Chŏngdong, trans. *Sinch'an kajŏnghak*, 7–12.

99. Consulting a physician trained in biomedicine was a lesson in GGK-published ethics textbooks as well. "Superstition," Lesson 12, Grade 4 (1922).

100. Exercise was the exception, as moral textbooks illustrated physical activity in schools.

101. This was also the case in the United States. Leaders in the American domestic science movement, Ellen Richards and Marion Talbot, asserted

in 1887 that "a knowledge of sanitary principles should be regarded as an essential part of every woman's education." Nancy Tomes, *The Gospel of Germs: Men, Women, and the Microbe in American Life* (Cambridge, MA: Harvard University Press, 1998), 135.

102. It is interesting to note in the *Ch'ejo* textbook, that teachers were instructed to pay special attention to the posture of female students even at play. While it is not stated in the manual why the posture of only girls and not boys is singled out, one possibility is that this overlaps with concerns for women's body alignment and reproductive health as seen in debates on women's clothing (particularly the deleterious effects of bindings) and physical education in Korean print media. Similar concerns over women's bodies circulated in Japan at this time. Yuki Terazawa, "Gender, Knowledge, and Power: Reproductive Medicine in Japan, 1790–1930" (PhD diss., University of California, Los Angeles, 2001).

103. Sarah Stage, "Introduction: Home Economics, What's in a Name?" in *Rethinking Home Economics: Women and the History of a Profession*, ed. Sarah Stage and Virginia B. Vincenti (Ithaca, NY, and London: Cornell University Press, 1997), 6.

104. Ava B. Millam, Dean of the Department of Domestic Science at Oregon Agricultural College (OAC), visited Ewha and helped start a scholarship fund for Asian students to study at OAC. She was in discussion with missionary Harriet Palmer Morris, a graduate of home economics at Kansas State Agricultural College, who was appointed to Ewha in 1921 and was instrumental in the establishment of Ewha's home economics (*kasa*) department at the college level. *Kajŏng kwahak taehak 70 nyŏnsa*, 10. Chemistry, natural studies (botany, zoology), and biology, for example, found practical application in food chemistry, nutrition, pharmacology, and basic nursing. Millam was dean when OAC began its "Practice House" to teach infant care, a model that Ewha subsequently adopted.

105. See Yukako Tatsumi, "Constructing Home Economics in Imperial Japan" (PhD diss., University of Maryland, College Park, 2011).

106. Yung-sik Kim, "Specialized Knowledge in Traditional East Asian Contexts," *EASTS* 4, no. 2 (2010): 180. For more on the history of science and technology in Korea, see Park Seong Rae, *Science and Technology in Korean History: Excursions, Innovations, and Issues* (Fremont, CA: Jain Publishing Company, 2005).

107. Although not stated here, this would be in contrast to cosmological expositions of the natural world as understood by Confucian scholars. *Sohakkyo kyoch'ik taegang* [Summary of the primary school regulation], 1895 as cited in Pak Chongsŏk, *Kaehwagi Hanguk ŭi kwahak kyogwasŏ* [Science

textbooks of Korea during the Enlightenment period] (Seoul: Hanguk haksul chŏngbo, 2007), 41.

108. Yi Myŏnu, "Kŭndae kyoyukki (1876–1910) hakhoejirŭl t'onghan kwahak kyuyuk ŭi chŏngae" [Science education through journals of academic societies 1876–1910], *Journal of Korean Earth Science Society* 22, no. 3 (2001): 85.

109. "Chehak sŏngmyŏng chŏryo" [Urgent explication of various studies], *Sŏbuk hakhoe wŏlbo* 11 (1909): 8–11.

110. Pot'ong hakkyoryŏng sihaeng kyuch'ik, 1906. As cited in Pak Chongsŏk, *Kaehwagi Hanguk ŭi kwahak kyogwasŏ*, 42. The 1929 GGK revisions to its educational policy officially categorized the various industrial and handicraft courses as *chigŏpkwa* or "the subject of vocational training." Kang Myŏngsuk, "Ilche sidae pot'ong hakkyo 'chigŏp' kyogwa ŭi toip kwa kŭ sŏnggyŏk" ["Vocational" subjects in normal school during the Japanese colonial period], *Kyoyuk sahak yŏngu* [Study of history of education] 21, no. 2 (2011): 8.

111. "Instructions Concerning the Enforcement of the Chosen Educational Ordinance," November 1, 1911, *Manual of Education in Chosen*, Appendix 12. Reprinted in *Singminji Chosŏn kyoyuk chŏngch'aek saryo chipsŏng*, vol. 2 (Seoul: Taehaksŏwŏn, 1990).

112. Article VI, Chapter II, "Regulation for Common Schools," October 20, 1911, *Manual of Education in Chosen*, Appendix 25.

113. Many went to Japan for further studies in the sciences. Keijō Imperial University, which opened in Seoul in 1924, had colleges only in law, medicine, and literature. For more on higher science education in colonial Korea, see Kim Kŭnbae, *Hanguk kŭndae kwahak kisul illyŏk ŭi ch'ulhyŏn* [The emergence of Korean modern science-technical manpower] (Seoul: Munhak kwa chisŏngsa, 2005).

114. "Instructions Concerning the Enforcement of the Chosen Educational Ordinance," November 1, 1911, *Manual of Education in Chosen*, Appendix 12.

115. *Manual of Education in Chosen*, 25.

116. Article XII, Chapter II, "Regulations for Common Schools," *Manual of Education in Chosen*, Appendix 30.

117. Information here is derived from the 1911 Educational Ordinance, various proclamations or instructions regarding this ordinance, and a table of curriculums for a common school. Reprinted in *Manual of Education in Chosen*, Appendix 1–39.

118. Article XII, Chapter II, "Regulations for Common Schools," *Manual of Education in Chosen*, Appendix 30.

119. "Instructions Concerning the Enforcement of the Chosen Educational Ordinance," November 1, 1911, *Manual of Education in Chosen*, Appendix 13.

120. Article XVII, Chapter II, "Regulation for Common Schools," October 20, 1911, *Manual of Education in Chosen*, Appendix 32.

121. Article XVIII, Chapter II, "Regulations for Girls' High Schools," October 20, 1911, *Manual of Education in Chosen*, Appendix 63.

122. "Instructions Concerning the Enforcement of the Chosen Educational Ordinance," November 1, 1911, *Manual of Education in Chosen*, Appendix 13.

123. Article XVII, Chapter II, "Regulations for Girls' High Schools," October 20, 1911, *Manual of Education in Chosen*, Appendix 63.

124. This conclusion is based on tables of contents of several *kaji* textbooks such as *Kindai kaji fuen shiryō shūsei* (Tokyo: Bunkōsha, 1932). These units are in line with GGK regulations that *kasa* provide "instruction in clothing, food and habitation, caring for the old and upbringing of children, nursing of the sick, cooking and other matters concerning house-keeping." Article XVII, Chapter II, "Regulations for Girls' High Schools," October 20, 1911, *Manual of Education in Chosen*, Appendix 63. Unfortunately, *kasa* textbooks were not preserved with the same care or interest as ethics, language, or history textbooks. Moreover, it is difficult to gauge which textbooks were used. Analysis of *kasa* textbooks comes from those on the approved list of the GGK and archived at Ewha Womans University's library.

125. Article IX, Chapter II, "Regulations for Girls' High Schools," October 20, 1911, *Manual of Education in Chosen*, Appendix 59.

126. One literary example where we see how a female student could deploy her skills learned in high school for paid employment is from Na Hyesok's 1918 story "Kyŏnghŭi," where the protagonist earns a wage sewing with machines at a textile factory.

127. "Instructions Concerning the Enforcement of the Chosen Educational Ordinance," November 1, 1911, *Manual of Education in Chosen*, Appendix 14.

128. The 1911 regulations for Girls' High School mandated 12–14 hours a week out of 31 total for science, *kasa*, sewing and handicrafts. In 1919, the number of hours were reduced to 9–11. Kang Tŏkhŭi, "Ku Hanmal kaehwagi put'ŏ 8.15 Kwangbok kkaji ŭi kajŏnggwa kyoyuk e kwanhan yŏngu" (PhD diss., Hanyang University, 1993), 71–72.

129. "Explanatory Statement on the Revision of the Regulations for High Schools and Girls' High School," *Manual of Education in Chosen*, Appendix 83.

130. This was a point raised by Jen-Der Lee at the International Conference on "The Making of 'Asia': Health and Gender," March 9–10, 2012, The University of Hong Kong.

131. Note, child-rearing was not taught at the elementary school level.

132. *Kindai kaji fuen shiryō shūsei* (Tokyo: Bunkōsha, 1932), 214–215. Not all *kasa* textbooks included information on the menstrual cycle.

133. This relates to a discourse in colonialist literature that the white clothing of Koreans was unhygienic and reflected their propensity for uncleanliness. See Todd Henry, "Sanitizing Empire." Interestingly, missionary Rosetta S. Hall made the opposite case, arguing for the better hygienic condition of white clothing.

134. *Kasa* textbooks were divided into two volumes, following Shimoda Utako's model. The first volume covered the units on clothing, food, and habitat. The second covered caring for the elderly, nursing, child-rearing, household economy, and household management. Chŏn Migyong, "Singminji sidae 'Kasa kyogwasŏ' e kwanhan yŏngu: 1930 nyŏndaerŭl chungsimŭro" [Analysis of household textbooks for middle high school in the colonial age], *Hanguk kajŏnggwa kyoyukhak hoeji* [Journal of Korean Home Economics Education] 16, no. 3 (2004): 15.

135. "The Caroline A. Ladd Hospital, of the Presbyterian Church in USA, Korea Mission, Pyongyang, Korea," *The Korean Mission Field* 5, no. 2 (1909): 25–29.

136. Harry A. Rhodes, "Presbyterian Theological Seminary," *The Korea Mission Field* 6, no. 6 (1910): 149–152.

137. Im Chŏngbin, "Kaehwagi Hanguk kajŏng saenghwal: *Maeil sinbo* sasŏl ŭl chungsimŭro" [Korean family life in early 20th century: Editorials of *Maeil sinbo*], *Hanguk kajok chawŏn kyŏngyŏnghak hoeji* 3, no. 1 (1999): 1–10.

138. Female physician Hŏ Yŏngsuk, for example, wrote a women's health column in *Tonga ilbo* from 1925.

139. As gathered from statistics cited from Kim Puja, *Hakkyo pak ŭi Chosŏn yŏsŏngtŭl*, 91.

140. Ibid., 92.

141. Pak Sŏnmi, *Kŭndae yŏsŏng cheguk ŭl kŏch'yŏ Chosŏn ŭro hoeyuhada, singminji munhwa chibae wa Ilbon yuhak* (P'aju, South Korea: Ch'angbi, 2007).

142. Ewha started the department in December 1928 but did not receive GGK accreditation until 1929.

143. *Kajŏng kwahak taehak 70 nyŏnsa*, 20.

144. Kim Hamna, "The Need of Home Economics Education in Korea," *The Korea Mission Field* 25, no. 10 (1929): 215–216.

145. Citizenship as cultural ideal stems from "What Does it Mean to be a Citizen?" *The Hedgehog Review* 10, no. 3 (2008): 5.

CHAPTER 2: FROM THE *ŬINYŎ* TO THE *YŎ'ŬI*

1. H. N. Allen, *First Annual Report of the Korean Government Hospital* (Yokohama: B. Meiklejohn & Co., 1886), reprinted in *Sources of Korean Christianity, 1832–1945*, ed. Sung-Deuk Oak (Seoul: The Institute for Korean Church History, 2004), 142.

2. See Allen's entry for August 5, 1886, in Horace Allen, *Allen ŭi ilgi* [Horace Allen's diary], trans. Kim Won-jo (Seoul: Dankook University Press, 1991), 478.

3. RSH (Rosetta Sherwood Hall), "The Past of Medical Missions in Korea," *The Korea Mission Field* 10, no. 7 (1914): 216–219. Ellers left medical work when she married a fellow missionary, the Reverend D. A. Bunker. Horton too left her position after her marriage to missionary Horace Underwood, but continued to practice medicine privately.

4. There are some discrepancies in sources in terms of the naming of Pogunyŏgwan (House for Caring and Saving Women). It is generally understood that it was granted its name by the queen, while other sources indicate that it was the king. Yi Pangwŏn, "Pogunyŏngwan ŭi sŏllip kwa hwaltong" [The establishment and activities of Pogunyŏgwan], *Ŭisahak* 17, no. 1 (2008): 37–56.

5. The East Gate Women's Hospital and its training of female medical personnel evolved into Ewha's Colleges of Nursing and Medicine after 1945.

6. Mrs. Theresa Ludlow, "Is it Worthwhile to Train Korean Nurses?" *The Korea Mission Field* 15, no. 10 (1919): 217–218.

7. M. J. Edmunds observes that young widows were the best candidates for nurse training, but even then the training of Korean nurses was challenging. M. J. Edmunds, "Training Native Nurses," *The Korean Mission Field* 2, no. 8 (1906): 154.

8. This contrasts with the 172 Japanese midwives and 220 Japanese nurses registered in Korea. GGK statistics come from *Chōsen sōtokofu tōkei nenpō* [Statistical yearbook of the Government-General in Korea]. Throughout the rest of the colonial period, the GGK did not distinguish between male and female physicians in its statistics so it is unknown how many total female physicians there were at a given time. However,

we do know that by 1910 only one Korean woman, Esther Pak (Kim Chŏmdong), was trained in biomedicine and worked as a physician in the new hospitals.

9. Other occupations mentioned in the article include reporter, kindergarten teacher, broadcast announcer, and telephone operator. "Yŏja chigŏp annae, ton ŏpsŏsŏ woeguk yuhak motgago ch'wijik hal kossŭn myŏtch'ina toenŭnga" [Survey of women's occupations, what jobs are available for those without the means to study abroad?], *Pyŏlgŏngon* 5 (1927): 100.

10. The monthly income of a midwife or physician would depend on how successful her private practice was, or if she was employed by a hospital, the salary determined by the hospital. A profitable private practice, it was claimed, could bring in as much as one hundred yen.

11. Aristocratic privilege through bureaucratic eligibility may have been conferred but not necessarily guaranteed by birth. Bureaucratic achievement (i.e., appointments, promotions) along with marriage patterns and wealth could affect lineage status and access to political power over time.

12. *Chungin* physicians working for the state were titled either *ŭiwŏn*, a general term for physician, or the more prestigious title *ŭigwan*, reserved for higher-ranked state physicians.

13. Kim Ho, *Hŏ Chun ŭi* Tongŭi pogam *yŏngu* [Study of Hŏ Chun's *Tongŭi pogam*] (Seoul: Ilchisa, 2000). A practitioner of *yangban* status would not be called *ŭiwŏn*.

14. For more on the *ŭinyŏ* system, see Hanguk yŏja ŭisahoe, *Hanguk yŏja ŭisa 90 nyŏn* [Korean female physicians, 90 years] (Seoul: Ŭihak ch'ulp'ansa, 1986); An Sanggyŏng, "Chosŏn sidae ŭi ŭinyŏ chedo e kwanhan yŏngu" [A study on the *ŭinyŏ* system in the Chosŏn dynasty] (PhD diss., Kyŏngsan University, 2000); Kim Miŭn, "Chosŏn sidae ŭinyŏ chedo e kwanhan koch'al" [Study of the Chosŏn period *ŭinyŏ* system] (MA thesis, Kyŏngsŏng University, 2004); and Pak Sŏnmi, "Chosŏn sidae ŭinyŏ koyuk yŏngu, kŭ yangsŏng kwa hwaldong ŭl chungsimŭro" [A study of education of *ŭinyŏ* during the Chosŏn period, their development and activity] (PhD diss., Chungang University, 1994).

15. For example, according to Yu Hŭich'un's sixteenth-century diary, "Miam ilgi," an *ŭinyŏ* was called in to attend to his wife and daughter but their medications were prescribed by a male *ŭiwŏn*. Sin Tongwŏn, "Chosŏn hugi ŭiyak saenghwal ŭi pyŏnhwa: sŏnmul kyŏngje esŏ sijang kyŏngje ro, 'Miam ilgi,' 'Soe mirok,' 'Yichae nango,' 'Hŭmyŏng' ŭi punsok" [Shift in everyday medical practices; from gift economy to market economy], *Yŏksa pip'yŏng* 75 (2006): 353.

16. One such highly skilled *ŭinyŏ*, *Changgŭm*, provided the inspiration for the long-running, high-grossing, and widely popular Korean TV series *Jewel in the Palace* (*Tae Changgŭm* MBC, 2003–2004).

17. The *kisaeng* were technically government slaves, selected, trained, and registered by the state to perform various official functions including needlework and entertainment with music and dance. Their association with leisure culture and illicit sexual relations belied their accomplishments in the fine, literary, and performing arts.

18. These practitioners were typically engaged in activities related to pharmaceutics more so than extensive diagnoses or therapeutics. Sin Tongwŏn, "Chosŏn hugi ŭiyak saenghwal ŭi pyŏnhwa," 364.

19. Midwifery as a formal profession did not exist in Korea before the twentieth century as it did in some European countries and Japan. Obstetrics was an essential part of the training of *ŭinyŏ* who took on an obstetrics-related role when working with women in the palace or elite families.

20. Ki Ch'angdŏk, "Kaehwagi ŭi Tongŭi wa Tongŭihak kangsŭpso" [Oriental medical doctors and the Oriental Medical Training Institute during the Enlightenment period], *Ŭisahak* 2, no. 2 (1993): 178–196. Such competition could grow fierce, however, when traditional practitioners deemed their livelihoods under threat. The animosity of human variolation inoculators toward the new state-dispatched smallpox vaccinators, for example, sometimes resulted in violent assaults on the latter. Sin Tongwŏn (Shin Dong-won), "Western Medicine, Korean Government, and Imperialism in Late Nineteenth-Century Korea: The Cases of the Choson Government Hospital and Smallpox Vaccination," *Historia Scientiarum* 13, no. 3 (2004): 164–175.

21. Medicine was conventionally brewed from a concoction of various *materia medica* and then ingested in a tonic.

22. A pharmacist was defined as one who managed an apothecary and prepared medicinal formulations prescribed by a physician. A drug seller sold drugs on the market.

23. As translated in chapter two of So Young Suh, "Korean Medicine." Suh's chapter provides a more detailed account of the 1900 and 1913 regulations regarding the medical profession. Other requirements for physicians included the prescription of medicine according to symptoms based on warm and cold attributes of medicinal drugs and techniques of acupuncture and moxibustion in line with classical principles of replenishment and depletion.

24. *Hwangsŏng sinmun*, August 20, 1902.

25. Ibid., March 9, 1900.

26. The Japanese RG and GGK agendas in their health administrations are documented in Pak Yunjae, *Hanguk kŭndae ŭihak ŭi kiwŏn* [The origin of the Korean modern medical system] (Seoul: Hyean, 2005); Sin Tongwŏn, *Hanguk kŭndae pogŏn ŭiryosa*; and Todd Henry, "Sanitizing Empire," and *Assimilating Seoul*. The GGK would occasionally publish reports on its health administration in English with statistics to narrate a success story in the control of communicable diseases.

27. Foreign physicians too had to meet the same criteria. It is interesting to note that graduation from medical school in the United States did not automatically qualify one for a medical license as the United States and Japan did not share reciprocity. Douglas B. Avison, the son of the superintendent of Severance Hospital, Oliver Avison, and a pediatrician active in infant welfare work in colonial Seoul, received his medical training in Canada and was thus exempt from the GGK licensing exams. Sherwood Hall, the son of Presbyterian medical missionaries James Hall and Rosetta S. Hall, decided to attend medical school in England so as to avoid the licensing exam requirement in Korea. He later became a major figure in tuberculosis work in Haeju. See his autobiography, *With Stethoscope in Asia* (McLean, VA: MCL Associates, 1978).

28. Letter from Dr. Moffit to Dr. Baugh, May 12, 1931. United Presbyterian Church in the U.S.A. Commission on Ecumenical Mission and Relations, Secretaries Files: Korea Mission, 1903–1972, Record Group 140, Presbyterian Historical Society, Philadelphia, Pennsylvania. Hereafter, RG 140, PHS.

29. The GGK did not recognize medical schools in the United States as providing the qualification for its graduates to receive a license without examination.

30. Chōsen sōtokofu, *Tōkei nenpō*, 1925.

31. Pak Yunjae, *Hanguk kŭndae ŭihak ŭi kiwŏn*, 305. Maximum fees physicians could charge for consultation and hospitalization were stipulated.

32. Because there is no comparable English term, *ŭisaeng* will remain in its Romanized form. The English translation for *ŭisaeng* comes from Soyoung Suh, *Naming the Local*, 62.

33. So Young Suh, "Korean Medicine Between the Local and the Universal," 110–111.

34. These journals include *Hanbang ŭiyakkye*, *Tongŭi pogam*, *Tongsŏ ŭihakpo* *Tongsŏ yŏnguhoe wŏlbo*, *Chosŏn ŭihakkye*, and *Tongyang ŭiyak*. Chŏng Chihun, "Ilche sidae hanŭi haksul chapchi yŏngu" [Research on academic journals of oriental medicine in the era of Japanese imperialism], *Hanguk ŭisahak hoeji* 14, no. 2 (2001): 173–188. *Ŭisaeng* organizations also published study guides to the *ŭisaeng* licensing exams such as the booklet

Ŭisaeng sihŏm munje haedapjip [Solution manual for the *ŭisaeng* examination], which I found in the archives of Dong-Eun Medical Museum at Yonsei University College of Medicine.

35. Yŏ Insŏk, Pak Yunjae, Yi Kyŏngnok, and Pak Hyŏngu, "Hanguk ŭisa myŏnhŏ chedo ŭi chŏngch'ak kwajŏng—Hanmal kwa Ilche sidaerŭl chungsimŭro" [A history of the medical licensing system in Korea from the Taehan to Japanese colonial period], *Ŭisahak* 11, no. 2 (2002): 137–153.

36. Pak Yunjae, *Hanguk kŭndae ŭihak ŭi kiwon*, 318. Colonial Taiwan also had a dual-tier system of physicians that Michael Shiyung Liu labels as Category A and Category B physicians. However, the second-tiered Category B did not refer to practitioners of traditional Chinese medicine, but referred to Taiwanese physicians whose medical practice remained primarily clinical and practical, not research-oriented. See Michael Shiyung Liu, *Prescribing Colonization: The Role of Medical Practices and Policies in Japan-Ruled Taiwan, 1895–1945* (Ann Arbor: Association for Asian Studies, 2009).

37. Byong-Hee Cho, "The State and Physicians in South Korea, 1910–1985: An Analysis of Professionalization" (PhD diss., University of Wisconsin–Madison, 1988), 73.

38. After 1910, its students were transferred to the GGK Hospital Training Institute.

39. Major mission hospitals beside Severance included the aforementioned East Gate Women's Hospital, William James Hall Memorial Union Hospital in Pyongyang, and Taiku Presbyterian Hospital in Taegu.

40. In 1909, the Korean Red Cross Hospital re-emerged but only as fused with the Japanese Red Cross Hospital. Yi Kkonme and Hwang Sangik, "Uri nara kŭndae pyŏngwŏn esŏ ŭi kanho" [Nursing in Korea's modern hospitals], *Ŭisahak* 6, no. 1 (1997): 55–72.

41. Sin Tongwŏn, "Ilche ŭi pogŏn ŭiryo chŏngch'aek mit Hangugin ŭi kŏngang sangt'ae e kwanhan yŏngu" [A study on the policy of health services and health state of Koreans in the Japanese colonial state] (MA thesis, Seoul National University, 1986), 74.

42. The first charity hospitals were established in 1909 before annexation.

43. The GGK established charity hospitals throughout the country, which provided many Korean patients' first experience with biomedicine. Some were converted from already established Dōjinkai hospitals, others were entirely new institutions. By 1912, there were eighteen charity hospitals. Pak Yunjae, *Hanguk kŭndae ŭihak ŭi kiwŏn*, 252.

44. The asylum at Sorokdo was considered part of the charity hospital system and is operated today as Sorokdo National Hospital by South Korea's Ministry of Health and Welfare.
45. This hospital was the forerunner of today's premier Seoul National University Hospital.
46. Pak Yunjae, *Hanguk kŭndae ŭihak ŭi kiwŏn*, 280–281.
47. According to statistics gathered in *Kyŏngsŏng ŭihak chŏnmunhakkyo illam* [Catalogue of Keijō Medical College] by Ki Ch'angdŏk, no Japanese student graduated from the GGK Hospital Training Institute and the first graduating class of Japanese students at Keijō Medical College was in 1920. As cited in Ki Ch'angdŏk, *Hanguk kŭndae ŭihak kyoyuksa* [A history of modern medical education in Korea] (Seoul: Academia, 1995), 152.
48. Pak Yunjae, *Hanguk kŭndae ŭihak ŭi kiwŏn*, 280–281.
49. The dean at the GGK Hospital Training Institute recorded in his memoirs his concerns that educating too many Korean physicians would reduce the willingness of the Korean populace to consult Japanese physicians. Pak Yunjae, *Hanguk kŭndae ŭihak ŭi kiwŏn*, 280.
50. Byong-Hee Cho, "The State and Physicians in South Korea, 1910–1985," 79.
51. Pak Yunjae, *Hanguk kŭndae ŭihak ŭi kiwŏn*, 288.
52. Michael Shiying Liu, *Prescribing Colonization*.
53. Pak Yunjae, *Hanguk kŭndae ŭihak ŭi kiwŏn*, 289. The special track was abolished in 1922. Ki Ch'angdŏk, *Hanguk kŭndae ŭihak kyoyuksa*, 176.
54. Ki Ch'angdŏk, *Hanguk kŭndae ŭihak kyoyuksa*, 149.
55. This admission guideline was abolished in 1922. Pak Yunjae, *Hanguk kŭndae ŭihak ŭi kiwŏn*, 288.
56. Chōsen sōtokofu, *Tōkei nenpō*, 1920, as cited in Yi Ch'ungho, *Hanguk ŭisa kyoyuksa yŏngu* [History of the education of physicians in Korea] (Seoul: Hanguk charyowŏn, 1998), 173.
57. Chŏng Chunyŏng, "Singminji ŭihak kyoyuk kwa hegemŏni kyŏngjaeng: Kyŏngsŏng chedae ŭihakpu ŭi sŏllip kwajŏng kwa chedojŏk t'ŭkjingŭl chungsimŭro" [Medical education and competition for hegemony in colonial Korea: Establishment and characteristics of Keijō Imperial University Medical Department], *Sahoe wa hyŏnsil* 85 (2010): 197–237. This is at a time when the medical field in Japan looked to Germany as a source of advanced medicine. Germany was also a destination for aspiring Japanese students seeking academic degrees in medicine. Hoi-eun Kim, *Doctors of Empire: Medical and Cultural Encounters between Imperial Germany and Meiji Japan* (Toronto: University of Toronto Press, 2014).

58. When KIUMD took over the GGK Hospital, Keijō Medical College had to construct a new hospital for its clinical education.
59. As cited in Chŏng Chunyŏng, "Singminji ŭihak kyoyuk kwa hegemŏni kyŏngjaeng," 203.
60. Ki Ch'angdŏk, "Kyŏngsŏng cheguk taehakkyo ŭihakpu" [Medical department of Keijō Imperial University], *Ŭisahak* 1, no. 1 (1992), 64–82.
61. Sin Kyuhwan and Sŏ Honggwan, "Hanguk kŭndae sarip pyŏngwŏn ŭi paljŏn kwajŏng, 1885 nyŏn-1960 nyŏn kkaji" [The development of private hospitals in modern Korea, 1885–1960], *Ŭisahak* 11, no. 1 (2002): 94, 96.
62. Pak Yunjae, "Ilcheha ŭisa kyech'ŭng ŭi sŏngjang kwa chŏngch'esŏng hyŏngsŏng" [The growth of physicians and formation of their subjectivity under Japanese colonial rule], *Yŏksa wa hyŏnsil* 63 (2007): 163–189.
63. Other medical schools in Korea included the medical training institutes attached to the provincial hospitals in Pyongyang and Taegu founded in the 1920s, and later gained professional school status. Students chose to study abroad often in Japan and Germany. Ki Ch'angdŏk, *Hanguk kŭndae ŭihak kyoyuksa.*
64. The case was similar for colonial Taiwan. See Ming-Cheng M. Lo, *Doctors within Borders: Profession, Ethnicity, and Modernity in Colonial Taiwan* (Berkeley and Los Angeles: University of California Press, 2002).
65. Pak Yunjae, "Ilcheha ŭisa kyech'ŭng ŭi sŏngjang kwa chŏngch'esŏng hyŏngsŏng," 175.
66. Byong-Hee Cho, 85. "The State and Physicians in South Korea, 1910–1985," 85.
67. The 1919 Private Hospital Regulation stipulated that a hospital had to have at least ten hospital beds in a separate isolation ward for patients with contagious diseases. This regulation posed a heavy financial demand that limited the abilities of those interested in establishing private hospitals. Sin Kyuhwan and Sŏ Honggwan, "Hanguk kŭndae sarip pyŏngwŏn," 89.
68. Pak Yunjae, *Hanguk kŭndae ŭihak ŭi kiwŏn*, 267–274.
69. Pak Yunjae, "Ilcheha ŭisa kyech'ŭng ŭi sŏngjang kwa chŏngch'esŏng hyŏngsŏng."
70. Ibid.
71. Physicians also inspired literary and artistic critiques as being money-grubbing, self-centered, and unpatriotic. One example is Kim Tongin, "Ŭisa wŏnmangi, sinsa ŭi pi'ae," *Tonggwang* 32 (1932): 84–87. Perhaps one of the best-known scathing characterizations of colonial period Korean physicians is the story of Dr. Yi Injik in "Kapitan Ri" (1962) by Chŏn Kwangyong.

72. For example, Yi Kapsu, a physician trained in Germany, was a leading member of the Korean Eugenics Association.
73. Yŏ Insŏk and Yi Kyuch'ang, "Hansŏng ŭisahoe e taehayŏ" [On Seoul Physicians' Association], *Ŭisahak* 1, no. 1 (1992): 31–35.
74. Several people died after being injected with emetine by the sanitary police, ostensibly as a treatment for lung distoma. Colonial officials declared that the cold weather, and not the injections administrated by the Bureau of Sanitation, was to blame, sparking outrage from the Korean public. Pak [Park] Yunjae, "The 1927 Emetine Injection Incident in Colonial Korea and the Intervention Emetine incident," *Korea Journal* 50, no. 1 (2010): 160–177.
75. Caprio, *Japanese Assimilation Policies in Colonial Korea*, 90. Other scholarship on racial biometrics include Mark Caprio, "Abuse of Modernity: Japanese Biological Determinism and Identity Management in Colonial Korea," *Cross-Currents: East Asian History and Culture Review* 10 (2014), http://cross-currents.berkeley.edu/e-journal/issue-10, and Jin-Kyung Park, "Husband Murder as the 'Sickness' of Korea: Carceral Gynecology, Race, and Tradition in Colonial Korea, 1926–1932," *Journal of Women's History* 25, no. 3 (Fall 2013): 116–140. For Korean research on racial biometrics see Soyoung Suh, *Naming the Local*, 88–95.
76. Byong-Hee Cho, "The State and Physicians in South Korea, 1910–1985," 85.
77. Pak Yunjae, "Ilcheha ŭisa kyech'ŭng ŭi sŏngjang kwa chŏngch'esŏng hyŏngsŏng."
78. Ch'ang Haeja, "Yŏhaksaeng ege ŭihak yŏngu rŭl kwŏngo" [Encouraging female students to study medicine], *Taehan hŭnghakpo* 6 (1909): 22–27.
79. It is this diagnostic method that foreign observers labeled as "pulse-taking," associated with traditional Korean medicine.
80. Jin-kyung Park, "Picturing Empire and Illness: Biomedicine, Venereal Disease, and the Modern Girl in Korea under Japanese Colonial Rule," *Cultural Studies* 28, no. 1 (2014): 108–141.
81. This was recounted in the *Seoul Press*, reprinted as "Korean Women and Medicine," *The Korea Mission Field* 11, no. 9 (1915): 257–258.
82. There were apparently three medical schools for women in China and one in India.
83. She followed the American practice of changing her surname after her marriage. See "Ch'oech'o yŏŭi Pak Esther yŏsa sojŏn" [Short biography of the first female physician, Esther Pak], *Sin kajŏng* (November 1934), 85–87; *Fifty Years of Light* (Seoul: Woman's Foreign Missionary Society of the Methodist Episcopal Church, 1938); and Sherwood Hall, *With Stethoscope in Asia*.

84. For more on Chinese medical students who were officially appointed as medical missionaries to China, see Connie Shemo, *The Chinese Medical Ministries of Kang Cheng and Shi Meiyu, 1872–1937: On a Cross-Cultural Frontier of Gender, Race, and Nation* (Bethlehem, PA: Lehigh University Press, 2011).

85. Sherwood Hall wrote in his memoir that Park's early death inspired him to dedicate his life in the fight against tuberculosis. Sherwood Hall, *With Stethoscope in Asia.*

86. Rosetta S. Hall and Mary Cutler "Kwanghyewŏn," 16th Annual Report to the Korea Woman's Conference (1914), 40–46. Hereafter, Korea Woman's Conference will be denoted by KWC.

87. Rosetta S. Hall, "Woman's Hospital of Extended Grace, Pyeng Yang," *The Korea Mission Field* 8, no. 8 (1912): 245–249.

88. Rosetta Sherwood Hall, "Women Physicians in the Orient," *The Korea Mission Field* 21, no. 2 (1925): 41.

89. Teacher training programs used to be handled by individual higher common schools for girls before the GGK consolidated teacher training in the Women's Department of the GGK Teacher Training School in 1925. Ewha gained GGK professional school status for its college in 1925.

90. Esther Pak practiced at a time before the GGK's 1913 Regulation for Physicians.

91. Rosetta S. Hall and Mary Cutler "Kwanghye yŏwŏn," *Annual Report of the Korea Women's Conference* (1914): 40–46. [Hereafter, *KWC*]

92. Dr. Rosetta Sherwood Hall, "The Woman's Medical Training Institute, Ella Anthony Lewis' Memorial, Seoul," *The Korea Mission Field* 24, no. 9 (1928): 182–183.

93. "Pyeng Yang Woman's Hospital of Extended Grace," *KWC* (1917): 110.

94. Rosetta S. Hall, MD, and Mary M. Cutler, MD, "Koang Hyoe Nyo Won" [Woman's Hospital of Extended Grace], 97–100.

95. "Dr. Hall's Report for the Year 1922," *KWC* (1923): 74.

96. "Haewoe haenae e hŏt'ŏsŏ itnŭn Chosŏn ŭisa p'yŏngp'angi," *Pyŏlgŏngon* 5 (1927): 70–74.

97. Ibid.

98. Rosetta Sherwood Hall, "Women Physicians in the Orient," 41.

99. The institutions at which these graduates practiced were Chemulpo Women's Hospital, Seoul Women's Hospital, East Gate Women's Hospital, and the infant welfare clinic at the Social Evangelistic Center. A few had private practices.

100. Ch'oe Ŭngyŏng, "Ilche kangjŏmgi Chosŏn yŏja ŭisadŭl ŭi hwaltong— Tokyo yŏja ŭihakkyo chorŏp 4 inŭl chungsimŭro" [The activities of

women physicians in colonial Korea—focusing on four graduates of Tokyo Women's Medical College], *Cogito* 80 (2016): 287–316.

101. Rosetta Sherwood Hall, "Women Physicians in the Orient," 41.
102. *Sin kajŏng* (March 1933): 118
103. Rosetta Sherwood Hall, "Women Physicians in the Orient," 41.
104. Ibid., 43.
105. *Tonga ilbo*, June 8, 1934. This article lists six graduates. However, the first issue (1934) of the school journal *Kyo'u hoeji*, states there were five graduates in 1934.
106. *Chosŏn chungang ilbo*, June 18, 1936.
107. Kil Chŏnghŭi, *Na ŭi chasŏjŏn*, 28–30. One should be mindful when reading her memoir given that she penned it decades after the colonial period. However, many of her statements on her motivations and reasons to enter the medical field resound with sentiments female physicians expressed in the print media and the Training Institute association's bulletin *Kyo'u hoeji*. The historiography of the Women's Medical Training Institute is divided generally into two camps—one that places missionaries and Rosetta S. Hall as main figures in the establishment of the school and the other that emphasizes it as an indigenous or Korean national achievement. Kil was proud of how the Training Institute was about to send out five to six female physicians "every year with our own strength." Kil's other main concern is that her husband be recognized for his continued support of the Training Institute despite being thwarted from being on its faculty due to the prison record that had led to his expulsion from medical school.
108. Kim Sangdŏk, "Yŏja ŭihak kangsŭpso, 1928 nyŏn esŏ 1938 kkaji" [The woman's medical training institute], *Ŭisahak* 2, no. 1 (1993): 81. Kim argues that the change in name highlights the colonial relationship between Korean reformers and their Japanese rulers. The name Chosŏn, which indicated the national identity of the school, was to be stripped and replaced with Kyŏngsŏng (Keijō), the Japanese imperial name for the Korean capital. This also followed the Japanese convention of naming an educational institution after the city in which it was located.
109. "Kyo'u hoegirok" [Minutes of the Kyo'uhoe], *Kyo'u hoeji* 1 (1934): 53.
110. Members of the committee included Yun Ch'iho, Helen Kim, and Pak Yŏnghyo. "Chaedan pŏbin yŏja ŭihak chŏnmun hakkyo palgi chunbi wiwŏnhoerok" [Minutes of the organizing committee for a women's medical college], *Kyo'u hoeji* 1 (1934): 54–56. I could only find one extant copy of the inaugural issue of *Kyo'u hoeji*. While this issue called for submissions for the second issue, none of the major archives in Korea, including the National Library, Seoul National University Library, which houses

the former library from Keijō Imperial University, Yonsei Library, Ewha Womans University, or Korea University had any other issue.

111. Kil Chŏnghŭi, *Na ŭi chasŏjŏn*, 35.
112. Ki Ch'angdŏk, "Sarip yŏja ŭihak kyoyuk" [The early history of private education of Western medicine for women], *Ŭisahak* 1, no. 2 (1993): 94.
113. Ki Ch'angdŏk, *Hanguk kŭndae ŭihak kyoyuksa*, 352, 356–357.
114. Pak Sŏnmi places the number at 103. *Kŭndae yŏsŏng, cheguk ŭl kŏch'ŏ Chosŏn ŭro hoeyuhada*], 50. Ki Ch'angdŏk gives a figure of 101 Korean female medical students in Japan, compared to 268 male students. Ki Ch'angdŏk, *Hanguk kŭndae ŭihak kyoyuksa*, 334.
115. The devastating damage caused by the earthquake and its aftershocks was compounded by rumors that Japanese suffered additional losses due to Korean culpability and criminal behavior (like poisoning wells). This sparked panic and a massacre of Koreans living in Tokyo. Fearing for her life, Kil stayed in her room for days but discovered her Japanese roommate felt suspicious and had reported Kil. Kil Chŏnghui, *Na ŭi chasŏjŏn*, 19.
116. Ch'oe Ŭngyŏng, "Ilche kangjŏmgi Chosŏn yŏja ŭisadŭl ŭi hwaltong.
117. "Yŏ'ŭi chwadamhoe" [Roundtable discussion among female physicians], *Sin kajŏng* (November 1934): 35–45.
118. For example, the numbers of dead due to contagious disease were recorded according to the illness, month of their death, age (in five-year spans) at death, and the province or even district of their death. "Restricted" license refers to a temporary license that permitted its holder the practice of medicine only to a limited space for a finite time.
119. Rosetta Sherwood Hall, "Women Physicians in the Orient," 41.
120. "Yŏ'ŭi chwadamhoe."
121. Son Ch'ijŏng, "Yŏŭirosŏ kkumkkunŭn yŏŭi chonghap pyŏngwŏn," *Sin kajŏng* (January 1935).
122. *Kyo'u hoeji* 1 (1934): 86–87.
123. Son Ch'ijŏng, "Yŏŭirosŏ kkumkkunŭn yŏŭi chonghap pyŏngwŏn."
124. Whether the position was temporary by design of the position or employer, or whether the women left their positions is unclear.
125. "Haewoe haenae e hŏt'ŏsŏ itnŭn Chosŏn ŭisa p'yŏngp'angi," *Pyŏlgŏngon* 5 (1927): 70–74.
126. "Interview of Dr. HJ," *Sanbuingwa ŭisa kusul charyo*. Name is not revealed to protect her identity. This comes from an unpublished collection of oral testimonies of obstetrician-gynecologists in the archives of the Institute for the History of Medicine, Yonsei University. Hereafter,

transcripts of these testimonies will be marked simply as *Sanbuingwa ŭisa kusul charyo*. The transcript of one interview was published in Yŏnse taehakkyo ŭihaksa yŏnguso, "Samil pyŏngwŏn sŏllipja, Yu Sŭnghŏn" [Founder of Samil Hospital, Yi Sŭnghŏn], *Yŏnsei ŭisahak* 12, no. 2 (2009): 59–103. I had the opportunity to work with the researchers on some of their interviews in 2009.

127. Rosetta Sherwood Hall, "Medical Work and Medical Education," *KWC* (1918, 1927, 1930).

128. "Yŏja chigŏp annae," 101.

129. "Naega pon na, myŏngsa ŭi cha-agwan," *Pyŏlgŏngon* 29 (1930): 57. Hŏ does return for further studies and medical work in the late 1930s.

130. Yi Sŏngun received his medical degree from Keijō Professional Medical School, worked in the GGK hospital and as a teaching assistant at the Keijō Imperial Medical University (1929–1933), before working at a municipal public hospital in Kyŏnggi Province and opening his own practice. He received his medical doctorate (PhD) from Kyushu Imperial University in 1941, and was a major figure in the medical field after 1945, working at Seoul National Medical University. His wife's name is anonymous in this article. Y reporter, "Haengbok toen kajŏng ŭl ch'ajŏsŏ: Pubuga moda ŭisarossŏ kŭllohanŭn haengbokdoen chip, so'agwa Yi Sŏngŭnssi kajŏng," *Yŏsŏng* (October 1938): 58–60.

131. "Ŭihak kangyŏnghoe kirok [Medical lectures]," *Kyo'u hoeji* 1 (1934): 79–80.

132. "Interview of Dr. HJ."

133. Haewoe haenae e hŏt'ŏsŏ itnŭn Chosŏn ŭisa p'yŏngp'angi," *Pyŏlgŏngon* 5 (1927): 70–74.

134. She did apparently help with her husband's private practice, which was run out of their home. Y reporter, "Haengbok toen kajŏng ŭl ch'ajŏsŏ."

135. She did not appreciate this about Yi. Hŏ Yŏngsuk, "Namp'yŏn'i malhanŭn annae ŭi hŏm, annaega malhanŭn namp'yŏn ŭi hŏm," *Pyŏlgŏngon* 33 (1930): 146–149.

136. "Yŏja chigŏp annae," 100–105.

137. Pak Sunjŏng, "Yŏsŏng ŭi kajŏng ŭihak" [Family medicine for women], *Kyo'u hoeji* 1 (1934): 16–25.

138. Chŏng Nami, "Uri yŏ'ŭigang ŭl sallija" [Let's save our Women's Training Institute], *Kyo'u hoeji* 1 (1934): 22–23.

139. Yu (Ryu) Yŏngjun, "Chosŏn ŭi yŏhakkyo" [Korea's girls' schools], *Kidok sinbo* (1926). As cited in Ch'oe Ŭngyŏng, "Ilche kangjŏmgi Chosŏn yŏja ŭisadŭl ŭi hwaltong," 305.

140. Hyŏn Tŏksin, "Chosŏn e yŏbyŏngwŏn i p'ilyohan iyu" [Reason Korea needs women's hospitals], *Kidok sinbo* (1926). As cited in Ch'oe Ŭngyŏng, "Ilche kangjŏmgi Chosŏn yŏja ŭisadŭl ŭi hwaltong," 305.
141. Kil Chŏnghŭi, *Na ŭi chasŏjŏn*, 13.
142. "Yŏ'ŭi chwadamhoe," 45.

CHAPTER 3: THE HEAVENLY TASK OF NURSING

1. *Tonga ilbo*, January 22, 1924.
2. Ibid., January 25, 1924.
3. Ibid., February 27, 1921. T'aehwa later became a union center of the two Methodist denominations along with the Presbyterian Church of the United States of America. The fact that missionaries translated *T'aehwa yŏjagwan* into English as the "Social Evangelistic Center" as opposed to the literal translation, "T'aehwa Women's Center," attests to the center's primary purpose of evangelism. It was also the predecessor to the center known today as *T'aehwa kidokkyo sahoe pokchigwan*, or Taihwa Christian Community Center. For a fuller history of T'aehwa, see Yi Tŏkchu, *T'aehwa kidokkyo sahoe pokchigwan ŭi yŏksa: 1921–1993* [History of Taihwa Christian Community Center] (Seoul: T'aehwa kidokkyo sahoe pokchigwan, 1993).
4. Yi Kkonme, "Han Singwang: Hanguk kŭndae ŭi sanp'a ija kanhobu rosŏ ŭi sam" [The life and work of Han Singwang: A midwife and nurse of Korean modern times], *Ŭisahak* 15, no. 1 (2006): 107–119.
5. According to GGK statistics, there were 758 midwives, including Japanese, overall. Chōsen sōtokofu, *Tōkei nenpō*.
6. Edna Lawrence, "Report of Severance Union Training School for Nurses and Midwives, 1927–28," *Bulletin of Nurses' Association* 9 (1928): 5.
7. Severance Hospital had some male nurses in 1906, but began to introduce female nurses to work in male wards. "Severance Hospital," *The Korean Mission Field* 2, no. 5 (1906): 93–96. Nevertheless, even in the late 1920s, nursing was not a popular occupation for women in Hamhŭng Province in the north. Nurses there tended to be male. "Report of Canadian Mission Hospital Nurses' Training School, Hamheung, Korea," *Bulletin of the Nurses' Association* 13 (1929): 20–21. GGK regulations did not prohibit the training of male nurses, only the licensing of male nurses, and the author admitted that they were no longer to accept male nursing students.

8. G. H. Jones, "The Capping of the Nurses," *The Korean Mission Field* 3, no. 4 (1907): 49–50.

9. "Extracts from the Report of the Korea Mission of the Northern Presbyterian Church," *The Korean Mission Field* 4, no. 9 (1908): 133–141.

10. Esther Lucus Shields, "Nurses Training School," *The Korean Mission Field* 5, no. 5 (1909): 84.

11. This was due to the fact that Korean applicants did not meet the qualifications due to their lower educational achievements. Yi Kkonme, *Hanguk kŭndae kanhosa* [History of modern nursing in Korea] (Seoul: Hanul Academy, 2002), 51–53.

12. The sixteenth-century record *Yangarok* mentioned in chapter 1 is an example of a *yangban* grandfather recording the illnesses of and directing the treatment for his grandson. See also Kim Ho, "18 segi huban kŏgyŏng sajok ŭi wisaeng kwa ŭiryo" [Health and medicine of capital-based elite families during the late 18th century], *Sŏul hak yŏngu* 11 (1998): 113–144.

13. Yi Kkonme and Hwang Sangik, "Uri nara kŭndae pyŏngwŏn esŏ ŭi kanho" [Nursing in Korea's modern hospitals], *Ŭisahak* 6, no. 1 (1997): 55–72.

14. RSH (Rosetta Sherwood Hall), "Pioneer Medical Missionary Work in Korea," in *Within the Gate*, ed. Charles A. Sauer (Seoul: Korea Methodist News Service, 1934), 103–105, and "Training School for Nurses," 98. See also Cutler and Edmunds, "Po Ku Nyon Koan," *KWC* (1904): 10.

15. Lillias H. Underwood records in her memoir how missionaries trained Korean Christian male converts from all social statuses at the isolation hospital. As discussed in an earlier chapter, this is a shift as men of *yangban* families disdained medical work at the wane of the nineteenth century. Lillias H. Underwood, *Fifteen Years Among the Top-Knots* (Seoul: Kyung-in Publishing, Co., 1977). Reprint of 1904 publication by American Tract Society.

16. *Kojong sillok*, December 12, 1905. http://sillok.history.go.kr/inspection /inspection.jsp?mTree=0&id=kza_14212012_001&keyword=%E7%9C% 8B%E8%AD%B7

17. Yi Kkonme and Hwang Sangik, "Uri nara kŭndae pyŏngwŏn esŏ ŭi kanho."

18. "Severance Hospital," *The Korean Mission Field* 2, no. 5 (March 1906): 93–96.

19. Yi Kkonme, *Hanguk kŭndae kanhosa*, 35.

20. "Report of Canadian Mission Hospital Nurses' Training School, Hamheung, Korea," *Bulletin of the Nurses' Association* 13 (1929): 20–21. GGK regulations did not prohibit the training of male nurses, only the licensing

of male nurses, and the author admitted that they were no longer able to accept male nursing students.

21. G. H. Jones, "The Capping of the Nurses."
22. Miss M. J. Edmunds, "Training Native Nurses," *The Korea Mission Field* 2, no. 8 (June 1906): 154–155.
23. The care of sick family members, particularly parents-in-law, was one of a woman's duties in the household. I conjecture that the practice today of relying on patients' relatives in hospital care is a legacy from this earlier period, when the lack of nurses required that relatives share in the provision of health care in hospitals.
24. Miss M. J. Edmunds, "Training Native Nurses."
25. Mrs. W. B. Harrison, "Training Nurses in Korea," *The Korea Mission Field* 12, no. 1 (1916): 25–27.
26. *Maeil sinbo*, December 10, 1920.
27. Goro Achiwa, "Linda Richards in Japan," *The American Journal of Nursing* 68, no. 8 (1968): 1716–1719.
28. "Red Cross Society," *Pot'ong hakkyo haktongyong susinsŏ* 4 (1907), reprinted in *Kŭndae hakbu p'yŏnch'an susinsŏ*, ed. Pak Pyŏnggi and Kim Minjae, 485–486.
29. For example, in the 1922 editions, the "Philanthropy" lesson featuring Florence Nightingale was taught in Lesson 16, Grade 4 ethics (*susin*) textbook.
30. It was not until the post-1945 period that the current term *kanhosa* (看護師) was used to indicate nurse. *Kanhobu* was changed to *kanhowŏn* by the Republic of Korea in 1951. It was changed again in 1987 to *kanhosa*, "sa" meaning teacher or mentor as is used in *ŭisa* for physician, indicating the intent to imbue more respectability on a more gender-neutral profession.
31. "Regulation of Nurses," GGK Ordinance #154. Reprinted in Yi Kkonme, *Hanguk kŭndae kanhosa*, 229–231.
32. This would include study abroad in Japan. One former midwife, for example, recalls studying nursing abroad in Osaka. "Interview with CD." [Name is not revealed to protect her identity.] This comes from an unpublished collection of oral testimonies of midwives in the archives of the Institute for the History of Medicine, Yonsei University. Hereafter, transcripts of these testimonies will be marked simply as *Sanp'a kusul charyo*. The project was introduced in Yŏnse taehakkyo ŭihaksa yŏnguso, "Chosansa int'ŏbu chŏngni" [Overview of interviews with midwives, *Yŏnse ŭisahak* [Yonsei Journal of Medical History] 11, no. 2 (2008): 87–91.
33. Yi Kkonme, *Hanguk kŭndae kanhosa*, 127.

34. "Mrs. Theresa Ludlow, "Is it Worthwhile to Train Korean Nurses?" *The Korea Mission Field* 15, no. 10 (1919): 217–218.
35. Mrs. G. Napier, "At Grips with Cholera," *The Korea Mission Field* 17, no. 3 (1921): 63–65.
36. Chŏng Chongmyŏng, "Kanhobu saenghwal" [Everyday life of a nurse], *Sin yŏja* 2 (1920): 51.
37. Miss M. J. Edmunds, "Training Native Nurses."
38. Chŏng Chongmyŏng, "Kanhobu saenghwal."
39. "Kanhobu ŭi saenghwal—T'aehwa chinch'also Han Singwang yang" [Lifestyle of a nurse, Miss Han Singwang of T'aehwa clinic], *Tonga ilbo*, March 18, 1925.
40. As discussed in a previous chapter, the only medical school available for women in Korea did not open until 1928.
41. Yi Kkonme, *Hanguk kanhosa*, 112.
42. Ibid., 72–73.
43. Ibid., 74.
44. Ibid., 62.
45. Chŏng was a widowed mother of an infant who returned to her home after the death of her husband. Han had to support her family after her brother was imprisoned for his organizing activities during the nationalist March 1st 1919 movement. For lengthier biographies of these women, see Yi Kkonme, "Han Singwang" and "Ilche kangjŏmgi sanp'a Chŏng Chongmyŏng sam kwa taejung undong [Life and activism of Chŏng Chongmyŏng, a midwife during the colonial period]," *Ŭisahak* 21, no. 3 (2012): 551–592.
46. Literature on the development of new midwifery in Japan explains that the appellation "New Midwife" was used in juxtaposition to "Elderly Woman," an unlicensed birth attendant. The Elderly Woman was blamed by administrators for performing unregulated abortions and infanticide. The New Midwife was trained in biomedical obstetrics to oversee pregnancy to ensure safe delivery and recovery; the occupation was standardized by the 1899 Midwifery Ordinance. Julie Rousseau, "Enduring Labors: The 'New Midwife' and the Modern Culture of Childbearing in Early 20th Century Japan" (PhD diss., Columbia University, 1998).
47. The household manual *Kyuhap ch'ongsŏ* recommended that the mother-to-be choose a few women experienced in childbirth to aid her during her delivery. Paek Okkyŏng, "Chosŏn sidae ch'ulsan e taehan insik kwa silje" [A study on the thought and historical fact about birth during the Chosŏn dynasty], *Ewha sahak yŏngu* 34 (2007): 210.
48. Rosetta Sherwood Hall, "The Native Doctor in Korea and His Work," *The Postgraduate*, reprinted in *The Life of Rev. William James Hall, M.D.:*

Medical Missionary to the Slums of New York, Pioneer Missionary to Pyong Yang, Korea, ed. Rosetta Sherwood Hall (Seoul: Hanguk kidokkyosa yŏnguhoe, 1984), 183.

49. The Regulation for the most part followed Japan's 1899 Midwifery Ordinance.

50. According to Yuki Terazawa, in Japan midwife regulations allowed older midwives who lacked biomedical knowledge and training but were experienced in assisting deliveries to continue their practices. Terazawa suggests this was intended to eliminate indigenous healers who competed with the state for control of women's bodies. Terazawa, "Gender Knowledge, and Power: Reproductive Medicine in Japan, 1790–1930" (PhD diss., University of California, Los Angeles, 2001), 374. This was not included in the midwife regulations in colonial Korea as it did not have a tradition of formal midwives. The 1914 Regulation on Midwives in Korea, however, did not specify that all deliveries were to be overseen by a licensed midwife or physician. Many women continued to deliver babies at home with the assistance of family members or friends. Nor were there enough midwives to attend to most deliveries.

51. Physicians apparently could charge two to five yen for assistance in delivery, while midwives visiting women at home could charge thirty-five sen per visit. Chōsen sōtokofu keimu sōkanfu, *Chōsen eisei hōkishū* [Compilation of Chosŏn hygiene regulations] (Keijō, 1917), 47. It is unlikely that midwives adhered to this pay schedule. Oral testimonies among the *Sanp'a kusul charyo* claim that a fee of one *kama* of rice was standard during the colonial period. Other midwives note that oftentimes they did not charge for their services when a patient's finances prohibited it.

52. "Sanp'a mit kanhobu hapkyŏkja," *Tonga ilbo*, June 9, 1923. Han Singwang was another one of the three Koreans to receive (by exam) her midwifery license. Eleven were Japanese and four were foreigners.

53. The numbers shift again in the 1940s, skewed heavily on the side of nurses. This is likely due to concerted efforts by the GGK to recruit and train more Korean nurses.

54. They also could work for hospitals and make house calls as they saw fit.

55. Yi Kkonme, "Han Singwang."

56. Chŏng Chongmyŏng, "Pingung, t'ujaeng, kodok ŭi pansaeng" [Destitution, struggle, half life of solitude], *Samch'ŏlli* 2 (September 1929): 35, 50.

57. "Sin Ch'aeho puin pangmungi" [Visiting Sin Ch'aeho's wife], *Tonga ilbo*, December 12, 1928.

58. "Interview with CD," *Sanp'a kusul charyo.* Cows are highly prized commodities in South Korea, especially in rural areas.

59. She did not indicate the occupation of her grandfather.

60. By 1932, the number of Korean licensed midwives caught up with the number of nurses, and some years even exceeded the number of Korean licensed nurses. The number of nurses jumped again with the second Sino-Japanese War as the Japanese imperial state sought to increase medical personnel after 1939.

61. "Ton pŏri hanŭn yŏja chigŏp t'ambanggi" [Female occupations that earn money], *Tonga ilbo*, March 20, 1928.

62. "Sin Ch'aeho puin pangmungi" [Visiting Sin Ch'aeho's wife], *Tonga ilbo*, December 12, 1928.

63. "Interview with CD," *Sanp'a kusul charyo.*

64. "Ŭisa wa sanp'a rŭl tullŏssago pok'haengk'oja," *Tonga ilbo*, June 25, 1923.

65. Yi Kkonme, *Hanguk kundae kanhosa*, 71. The crash course ended in 1922, although it was occasionally resumed at the request of the police for their family members. This would suggest that the midwife crash course was intended not only for local surveillance purposes but also to offer educational and vocational opportunities for one's family while on duty in local areas.

66. Ibid., 55.

67. Ibid., 80.

68. "East Gate Women's Hospital," *Bulletin of the Nurses' Association of Korea* 11 (1928): 2. This report stated that schools had to require six years of elementary school and two years of higher education from its applicants to be considered for accreditation.

69. Sherwood Hall, "Pioneer Missionary Work in Korea," in *Within the Gate*, 98.

70. Some of the information presented here on foreign medical missions and infant welfare work first appeared in "Missionaries and 'A Better Baby Movement' in Colonial Korea," in *Divine Domesticities*, ed. Margaret Jolly and Hyaeweol Choi, 57–83. In chapter 4 and the epilogue, I revisit arguments on birth control and eugenics made earlier in "'Limiting Birth': Birth Control in Colonial Korea," *East Asian Science, Technology, and Society: An International Journal (EASTS)* 2, no. 3 (2008): 335–359. I am grateful to the Australian National University Press and Duke University Press for allowing me to incorporate material from those publications to support the current discussion in this book.

71. "Annual Report of 'In His Name Hospital,' Syen Chen (Sinch'ŏn), Korea, 1918–1919," RG 140, PHS.

72. R. K. Smith. "Medical Practice in Chosen," *The Korea Mission Field* 13, no. 5 (1917): 120–122.

73. A. G. Fletcher, "Concentration and Efficiency," *The Korea Mission Field* 12, no. 2 (1916): 39–44.

74. Even missionaries were not immune from the allure of other opportunities. For example, Dr. Wells, active in Pyongyang, resigned from the Presbyterian Mission in 1916 in order to work as a physician for the Seoul Mining Company. "The Resignation of Dr. and Mrs. Wells from the Presbyterian Missions, North," *The Korea Mission Field* 12, no. 1 (1916): 29. He was not the only one to do so. In 1909, another medical missionary resigned to work for the American Gold Mining Company. "Annual Report of Kwangju Station, Southern Presbyterian Mission," *The Korea Mission Field* 5, no. 4 (1909): 58–64.

75. W. E. Reid, "The Annual Meeting of the Korea Medical Missionary Association, Sept 30th to Oct 2nd, 1913, at Severance Hospital, Seoul," *The Korea Mission Field* 9, no. 12 (1913): 316–318.

76. "From the View Point of the Doctors," *The Korea Mission Field* 9, no. 2 (1913): 43–45.

77. W. E. Reid, "The Annual Meeting of the Korea Medical Missionary Association," 318.

78. Hugh H. Weir, M.D., "The Place of Medical Mission Work in Korea," *The Korea Mission Field* 10, no. 7 (1914): 191–193.

79. There apparently was dissatisfaction as the physician in charge (A. G. Anderson) was related to the nurse superintendent (Naomi Anderson), although there were plenty of Korean women to use as nurses. *Tonga ilbo*, November 25, 1921.

80. Interestingly, I have yet to locate mention of any disputes between mission hospital staff and Korean nurses and students in the mission archives. The closest comment I came across was a 1928 mention that, in 1926, the nursing training school at East Gate Women's Hospital did not accept a new class "due to various reasons." *Bulletin of Nurses' Association in Korea* 11 (1928): 4.

81. They apparently received eight to thirteen yen a month. *Tonga ilbo*, January 13, 1924. Missionaries have also admitted that they lost Korean medical personnel (including physicians) because of the lower salaries at mission hospitals.

82. *Tonga ilbo*, January 28, 1926.

83. Yi Kkonme, *Hanguk kŭndae kanhosa*, 188.

84. A Severance Hospital Nurses' Association was formed beforehand and met monthly for recreation or conferral. There was also an Association of Occidental Graduate Nurses that was organized in 1908, and later reorganized in the 1920s. *Bulletin of Nurses' Association in Korea* 1 (1925):

4. Also, in colonial Korea, the nursing associations included both nurses and nurse-midwives. After 1945, the nursing and midwifery professions were differentiated with separate organizations.

85. *Bulletin of Nurses' Association in Korea* 9 (1928): 20.

86. In its first year, there were twice as many foreign members as Korean.

87. In certain years, it published only one *Bulletin*. In other years, the KNA published 2–4 issues.

88. "Chosŏn kanhobu saŏp sangt'ae" [State of Korean nursing activities], *Chosŏn kanhobu hoebo* [Bulletin of the Nurses' Association in Korea] 14 (1929): 1–5. The title for the *Bulletin* will be given in Korean when the article is written in Korean and located in the Korean section of the *Bulletin*. When referencing articles printed in the English version of the journal, the English title of the *Bulletin* will be given.

89. *Bulletin of Nurses' Association in Korea* 2 (1926): 35.

90. Yi Kkonme, "Ilche sidae ŭi kanho tanch'e e kwanhan koch'al: Chosŏn kanhobuhoe ŭi kanho sujun hyangsang noryŏk kwa Chosŏn kanhobu hyophoe ŭi sahoe hwaltong" [A study of two nursing associations: Chosŏn kanhobuhoe's efforts to improve standards of nursing and the Chosŏn kanhohyŏphoe's societal concerns], *Kanho haengjŏnghakhoeji* 6, no. 3 (2000): 421–429. Interestingly, the Korean branch used the same name as that of the Nurses' Society founded by Han Singwang and others in 1924, which was no longer active.

91. The author argued that economic independence is the key to women's liberation, and jobs fitting women included teaching and clerical work. Women should consult parents or have chaperones in relations with men. Yi Yongsŏl, "Hyŏnsil uri Chosŏn yŏja ŭi todŏk p'yojun" [What kind of moral standard should we Korean women establish?], *Chosŏn kanhobu hoebo* 3 (1926): 6–10.

92. Kim Hyŏnmi, "Kyŏngsŏng Severance pyŏngwŏn esŏ kŭnmuhadŏn kanhowŏn ko Kim Sungyŏng yŏsa ŭi nangnyŏl" [In memory of nurse Kim Sungyŏng who worked at Severance Hospital in Seoul], *Chosŏn kanhobu hoebo* 3 (1926): 17.

93. Pang Kisun, "Kanho chingmu kajin urinŭn mu'ŏsŭl hanŭn kŏsi ollŭlka" [What should we do in our nursing roles?], *Chosŏn kanhobu hoebo* 5 (1927): 7–8.

94. During this period, mission hospitals increasingly depended on the services of Korean physicians, however. The East Gate Women's Hospital, for example, had Korean physicians on staff, and the public health and child welfare projects run by missionaries were also reliant on Korean physicians, nurses, and midwives.

95. *Bulletin of the Nurses' Association in Korea* 4 (1927): 16–17.

96. "Agi chŏt mŏginŭn pŏp kwa kirŭnŭn pŏp" [Feeding and care of infants], *Chosŏn kanhobu hoebo* 5 (1927): 10.

97. Han Singwang, "Chorŏpto handal pakke, kujikhanŭn irŭl wihaya (7)" [One month before graduation, for those looking for work], *Tonga ilbo*, March 18, 1925.

98. *Tonga ilbo*, July 4, 1825.

99. Ibid., July 21, 1925. The time from the March 1st movement in 1910 to the mid-1920s with the shift in colonial administration toward Cultural Rule, has been noted as a time of expanding publishing and social activities, as many of the heavy restraints on printing and assembly were relaxed. Leftist organizations were more openly active at this time before the crackdowns of the late 1920s made it extremely difficult to publicly express leftist opinions. Michael Robinson, *Cultural Nationalism in Colonial Korea, 1920–1925* (Seattle: University of Washington Press, 1988).

100. According to Yi Kkonme, when Han returned to Korea in 1927, she did not resume leadership or involvement with nursing organizations but turned her attention to women's social organizations such as the *Kŭnuhoe*. She was imprisoned a few months for her involvement in the 1928 Kwangju student movement. In the 1930s, Han left Seoul and social activism, running a midwifery practice in Masan. Yi Kkonme, "Han Singwang."

101. United States Children's Bureau and Nettie Pauline McGill, *Infant Work in Europe: An Account of Recent Experiences in Great Britain, Austria, Belgium, France, Germany, and Italy* (Washington, DC: U.S. Government Printing Office, 1921), 7.

102. An T'aeyun, *Singminji chŏngch'i wa mosŏng*.

103. A. F. Hillman, M.D., "Chong Dong Dispensary and Medical Work in Ewha Haktang, Seoul," *KWC* (1912): 54–56.

104. See annual reports of the Korea Woman's Conference of the Methodist Episcopal Church in the early 1900s.

105. "What Are You Doing in Your Station for the Help of Mothers, Especially in the Home and with Little Children?" *The Korea Mission Field* 12, no. 4 (1916): 114.

106. Mabel R. Genso, "Work with Korean Mothers," *The Korea Mission Field* 15, no. 12 (1919): 263–264.

107. Elma T. Rosenberger. "Public Health Work at the Social Evangelistic Centre, Seoul," *Bulletin of Korean Nurses' Association* 9 (1928): xv–xviii.

108. Elma T. Rosenberger, "Report of Public Health Work, Social Evangelistic Centre, Seoul," *Bulletin of Nurses' Association of Korea* 13 (1929): 28–31.

109. Clean, heated water as well as a large enough container to bathe in were luxuries that many Korean households did not have. Bathing was considered necessary to cleanliness, paramount in missionaries' understandings of health. Thus baths were common in infant welfare programs, although, in this case, they were aimed at bringing older street children into contact with the Center staff who would later visit their homes to evangelize. "Annual Report, Social Evangelistic Center, Seoul, Korea, January 1932," RG 140, PHS.

110. The soy formula was developed at Peking Union Medical College. At T'aehwa it was deemed to cost only three sen per feeding in contrast to the 10 sen for canned cream. N. Found, "A Cheap Substitute for Milk," *The China Medical Journal* 45, no. 2 (1931): 144–146. See also "Annual Report Social Evangelistic Center, Seoul, Korea, January 1932."

111. Kim Hamna, "The Need of Home Economics Education in Korea."

112. One example of the association's endorsed publications includes Frances Lee's *Children Nutrition and Health*. "Endorsed N.A.K. Publications," *Bulletin of the Nurses' Association in Korea* 24 (1932): 64–65.

113. "A Public Health Aeroplane Trip from North to South in Korea," *The Korea Mission Field* 36, no. 5 (1940): 81–83; and Maren P. Bording, "Infant Welfare and Public Health Work in Kongju," *The Korea Mission Field* 24, no. 3 (1928): 52–53.

114. A. G. Fletcher, "Concentration and Efficiency," 42.

115. See letter from Arthur J. Brown to Ms. Schauffler, October 19, 1925, RG 140, PHS. This was in fear that should support not be continued, the Mission Board did not want to be financially responsible for maintaining hospital operations.

116. Union work refers to different projects shared by Mission Boards from different denominations or even countries. Severance Hospital is an example of union work.

117. Dr. Douglas Avison noted, "[Child welfare clinics] take time, workers, and money. The work is enjoyable but when added to an already overload, they sometimes tax both patients and strength." See "Personal report of Douglas Avison, 1932–3," RG 140, PHS.

118. Soy milk formula was offered to poorer patients as an alternative.

119. "Report of the Cornelius Baker Memorial Hospital, Andong, 1930," RG 140, PHS.

120. Dr. Sharrocks explained that "Jesus Christ had compassion on the multitude" and commissioned that there be healing of the sick in the Church. A. M. Sharrocks, "Can Less Than Two Doctors in a Single Hospital Achieve the Best Result?" *The Korea Mission Field* 12, no. 1 (1916): 15–19.

121. William Ernest Hocking, *Re-thinking Missions: A Laymen's Inquiry after One Hundred Years* (New York and London: Harper and Brothers Publishers, 1926), 198–199.

122. "Kennedy Memorial Hospital Report, 1919–1920," RG 140, PHS.

123. J. D. Van Buskirk, "Christian Medical Education, Its Place and Opportunity," *The Korea Mission Field* 20, no. 7 (1914): 213–214.

124. E. W. Demaree, "The Future of Medical Missions in Korea," *The Korea Mission Field* 30, no. 4 (1934): 74–76.

125. O. R. Avison, "Social Service and the Hospital," *The Korea Mission Field* 20, no. 7 (1914): 203–206.

126. Hocking, *Re-thinking Missions*, 213.

127. "Public Health Institute," *Bulletin of Nurses' Association of Korea* 5 (1927): 5–13.

128. Ibid., 11.

129. Ibid., 12.

130. Ibid., 6.

131. Charles Sauer, *Within the Gate*, 105.

132. This is in contrast to other aspects of medical work where missionaries contested with the state, such as physician licensing, teaching credentials, and operation of smaller or less equipped clinics.

133. Esther L. Shields, "Mrs. Ludlow and Kim Whe Soon," *Bulletin of Nurses' Association* 3 (1926): 12–13.

134. Kim Hyegyŏng, *Singminjiha kŭndae kajok ŭi hyŏngsŏng chendŏ* [The formation of the modern family and gender during the colonial period] (Seoul: Ch'angbi Publications, 2006), 152.

135. Elisabeth S. Roberts, "Report of East Gate Hospital," *Bulletin of Nurses' Association of Korea* 13 (1929): 26–27.

136. Although mission sources indicate Lee received a degree from the University of Toronto, the Public Health program there has no record of her graduation. I did, however, find her name listed in a directory of students. It is likely that her study there was a result of an arrangement between the university and missionaries. Lee shared a room with a student from China who also was sponsored by missionaries. This was a period when the program in Public Health Nursing was being developed at the University of Toronto.

137. Personal report of Bertha Stanley Byram, 1928–29, RG 360, PHS.

138. Eva H. Field Pieters' letter dated January 4, 1931, RG 360, PHS.

139. One example is Ms. Ch'oe from Chŏnju whose articles appear in the *Kidok sinbo* in 1919 and 1920.

140. One example is Esther Koh (Ko Hwanggyŏng), who worked in mission social service centers during the colonial period and continued welfare work with women and children in the post-liberation period. She was the only woman to serve on a committee advising Park Chung Hee on family planning.

CHAPTER 4: NEGOTIATING GYNECOLOGY

1. The most common complaints were "medical," followed by "surgical." By "medical," Hall was likely referencing cases considered under general or internal medicine. Rosetta Hall and Esther Pak, "Woman's Medical Work, Pyeng Yang," *The Korean Mission Field* 5, no. 7 (1909): 109–111.
2. Mrs. Rosetta S. Hall, MD, and Miss Mary M. Cutler, MD, "Medical report of Pyeng Yang Hospital," *KWC* 17 (1915): 41–44.
3. "Pyeng Yang Woman's Hospital of Extended Grace," *KWC* 19 (1917): 105–112.
4. *Tonga ilbo*, September 15, 1924.
5. Kim Myŏnghŭi, "Sip'yŏng" [Comments on current events], *Sin yŏsŏng* 3, no. 1 (1925): 10–13.
6. Kim Miyŏng, "Ilcheha *Chosŏn ilbo* ŭi 'Kajŏng puinnan' yŏngu" [A study of the *Chosŏn ilbo*'s family wife column under Japanese colonial rule], *Hanguk hyŏndae munhak yŏngu* 16 (2004): 221–278.
7. Theodore Jun Yoo makes similar observations about the pathological nature of women's menstrual cycles in his book, *The Politics of Gender in Colonial Korea*. The pathological nature of women's bodies, as it is based on a biomedical understanding of the female anatomy, was not particular to Korea. Women's pathological nature can be seen in gynecological treatises in China as well as the West. See Frank Dikköter, *Sex, Culture, and Modernity in China: Medical Science and the Construction of Sexual Identities in the Early Republican Period* (Honolulu: University of Hawai'i Press, 1995).
8. Hŏ Sin, "Puinbyŏng ŭi chisik" [Understanding *puinbyŏng*], *Yŏsŏng* 4, no. 2 (1939): 56–59. Hŏ was employed as a physician by the GGK in various public hospitals before entering the obstetric-gynecological department of the teaching hospital of the medical department at Keijō Imperial University in the late 1920s. He also was a columnist for the *Tonga ilbo* and member of the Association of Korean Physicians (*Chosŏn ŭisa hyŏphoe*).

He eventually opened his own practice in 1932 and received a PhD from Keijō Imperial University in 1934. Sin continued to contribute women's health related articles to various journals throughout the 1930s and early 1940s.

9. According to Theodore Jun Yoo, *hwabyŏng* referred to what was perceived as the psychosomatic manifestation of the "accumulation of pent-up or unresolved anger over some kind of unjust social situation, which had built up for a long period of time." *It's Madness: The Politics of Mental Health in Colonial Korea* (Oakland: University of California Press, 2016), 39.

10. See the *puin* (wife/woman) chapter of the *chapbyŏng* (miscellaneous disease) section of the *Tongŭi pogam*.

11. Charlotte Furth, *A Flourishing Yin: Gender in China's Medical History, 960–1665* (Berkeley and Los Angeles: University of California Press, 1999), 55.

12. My mother, trained at Ewha's medical college in the 1960s, told me *puinbyŏng* referred to venereal disease. Dr. PP, a gynecologist whose interview is part of *Sanbuingwa ŭisa kusul charyo* gynecologist oral history project archived at the Institute for History of Medicine, Yonsei University, answered that *puinbyŏng* indicated infections or inflammations stemming from complications from tumors or cancer. This suggests how post-1945 biomedically trained or practicing physicians understood *puinbyŏng*.

13. Hŏ Sin, "Puinbyŏng ŭi chisik."

14. A survey concluded that women may live longer than men, but their quality of life was worse off as they were plagued by many diseases, *puinbyŏng* being among them. "Namja poda changsuhaedo pyŏngŭn yŏja e mana" [Although they live longer than men, women are more diseased], *Tonga ilbo*, September 26, 1931.

15. Charlotte Furth, *A Flourishing Yin*, 59.

16. Carroll Smith-Rosenberg and Charles Rosenberg, "The Female Animal: Medical and Biological Views of Woman and Her Role in Nineteenth-Century America," *Journal of American History* 60 (1973): 332–356.

17. Ann Douglas Wood, "'The Fashionable Diseases': Women's Complaints and Their Treatment in Nineteenth-Century America," *The Journal of Interdisciplinary History* 4 (1973): 25–52.

18. Richard Quain Bart, ed., *A Dictionary of Medicine: Including General Pathology, General Therapeutics, Hygiene, and the Diseases of Women and Children* (New York: D. Appleton and Company, 1895), 1237–1238.

19. Chang Mungyŏng, "Ch'ŏnyŏ p'ilyo tok ŭi wŏlgyŏng tokpon" [What young

women must read, a reader on menstrual cycle], *Sin kajŏng* (March 1936): 45–50.

20. See Kil Chŏnghŭi, "Wŏlgyŏng kwa wisaeng" [Menstruation and hygiene], *Yŏsŏng chi u* 1, no. 2 (1929): 56–57; Chŏng Kŭnyang, "Sŏng saengnihak, 2" [Sex physiology, 2], *Yŏsŏng* 1, no. 7 (1936): 36–37.

21. Changes a woman might experience during menopause, or that some of the symptoms of *puinbyŏng* might indicate cancer, may be mentioned in gynecology-related texts; however, they would not receive the same attention (preventive measures, instructions on care, causal factors, etc.) as *puinbyŏng* or other ailments that might affect women's reproductive functions such as venereal disease.

22. One was conducted by a Dr. Young-Chun Lee in Seoul in 1929, another much earlier in 1914 in Pyongyang by a Dr. Nigeda, Dr. J. W. Hirst at Severance in 1927, and another by Dr. Tchi-wang Yun also at Severance in 1931. Yun Ch'iwang, "Chosŏnin ŭi wŏlgyŏng ch'o chonyŏn ryŏng" [The age of onset of menstruation in Koreans], *Chosŏn ŭibo* 2, no. 2 (1931): 9–10. Soyoung Suh argues that research such as this was part of biometrics, or racial science, which sought to use scientific investigation to determine embodied differences of racialized bodies, in this case of Koreans. Soyoung Suh, *Naming the Local*, 88–95.

23. Wu Kok saeng, "Wŏlgyŏngnon" [Treatise on menstruation], *Yŏjagye* 3 (1918): 43–49.

24. "Yŏja ŭi kŏngang kwa wŏlgyŏng" [Women's health and menstruation], *Hyŏndae puin* 1 (1926): 16–18.

25. "Puinbyŏng ŭi iyagi" [About *puinbyŏng*], *Tonga ilbo*, August 31–September 3, 1927.

26. In the *ŭisaeng* journal *Tongsŏ ŭihak yŏnguhoe wŏlbo* [Monthly bulletin of the Association for Studying Eastern and Western Medicine], the Association for Studying Eastern and Western Medicine listed a chart that translated terms used for ailments in the Sino-classical medical tradition. *Taeha* here was correlated with the biomedical diagnosis *chagung naemak yŏm* or "endometrial inflammation." "Tongsŏ pyŏngmyŏng taejop'yo" [Chart of Eastern and Western disease terminology], *Tongsŏ ŭihak yŏnguhoe wŏlbo* 1, no. 1 (1923): 16–22.

27. Hŏ Chun and the *Tongŭi pogam* kugyŏk wiwŏnhoe [Committee on the vernacular translation of the *Tongŭi pogam*], *Tongŭi pogam* (Seoul: P'ungnyŏnsa, 1966).

28. An example is a series of articles on "uterine ailments" and pregnancy by Japanese obstetrician-gynecologist Kudō Takeshiro, director of Keijŏ

Women's Hospital in Seoul, in the publication of the Association for the
Study of Eastern and Western Medicine. Kudō's close ties to the colonial
government and his gynecological research on Korean female inmates
are analyzed by Jin-kyung Park, "Husband Murder as the 'Sickness' of
Korea."

29. This conclusion comes from my overview of the *ŭisaeng* journals extant at
Severance Hospital in Seoul and from secondary scholarship by Soyoung
Suh, Kim Nam-il, and Chŏng Chihun. See Chŏng Chihun, "Ilche sidae
hanŭi haksul chapchi yŏngu" [Research into academic journals of oriental medicine in the era of Japanese imperialism], *Hanguk ŭisahak hoeji*
14, no. 2 (2001): 173–188. Kim Nam-il, faculty of Kyunghee University's
College of Korean Medicine (*Hanŭi*), also has a blog on Korean Medicine
on the Korean Naver search engine site.

30. An example of this is the 1926 series on "Puingwa ch'ibyŏng yogyŏl" [Key
to treating gynecological diseases], in *Tongsŏ ŭihak*.

31. Kim Pyŏngha, "Imsin ojopyŏng e taehaya" [Ojo illness during pregnancy],
Hanbang ŭihak 11 (1913): 24–27.

32. Shiroda Bushi, "Purimjŭng ŭi ku ch'iryo e taehaya" [Treating infertility
with moxibustion], *Hanbang ŭihak* 11 (1913): 31–36.

33. Chang Mungyŏng, "Ch'ŏnyŏ ŭi p'ildok." This "alternate bleeding" appears
in both earlier Western and Sino-classical gynecological thinking. In the
West, vital fluids of the body needed releasing, and in Chinese medicine, excess Female Blood also needs releasing. How Chang explains this
within her description of menstrual bleeding as a shedding of the uterine
lining is unclear. Nevertheless, this indicates how earlier understandings
of the female body and processes persisted in newer biomedical models.

34. Kim Sŏghwan, "Chagung naemagyŏn, kyŏ-ul e manŭn naengbyŏng e
taehayŏ" [Infection of the uterine membrane, regarding *naeng* disease,
which is common in winter], *Chogwang* 2, no. 12 (1936): 333–337.

35. In other places, *naeng* was also used to translate "frigidity."

36. Cho Hŏnyŏng, "Puinbyŏng ŭi sŏbyang kwa ch'iryo (3)" [Care and treatment for *puinbyŏng*], *Ch'unch'u* (March 1944): 77–86. Cho (1900–1988)
is often portrayed in Korean medical scholarship as a Korean nationalist
who was active in nationalist organizations such as the Singanhoe, and
a strong advocate for Korean traditional medicine, having penned several treatises that sought its synthesis with biomedicine such as *T'ongsŏk
hanŭihak wŏllon* [Theory of Korean medicine] (1934) and *Puinbyŏng
ch'iryobŏp: yŏgwa chŭngch'i* [Treating women's disease: Symptoms and
treatment in gynecology] (1941). He was allegedly abducted to North

Korea after 1945, where he re-emerged as a major figure in Korean Medicine in the North. See Sin Ch'anggŏn, "Cho Hŏnyŏng ŭi chŏngch'ijŏk ŭihak sasang—singminjigi, haebang hu, 'nanbuk' hu rŭl t'onghayŏ" [Cho Heon-Yeong's political thought of medicine] *Hanguksa ron* 42: 115–151, and Pak Yunjae, "1930~1940 nyŏndae Cho Hŏnyŏng ŭi hanŭihak insik kwa tongsŏ chŏlch'ungchŏk ŭihangnon" [Jo Heonyeong's understanding of and vision for the future of Korean Traditional Medicine in the 1930–1940s], *Hanguk kŭnhyŏndaesa yŏngu* 40 (2007): 118–139, 260–261.

37. Pak Sŏkbin, "Kyŏ-ul kwa chilbyŏng, kyŏ-ul kwa puinbyŏng" [Winter and disease, winter and *puinbyŏng*], *Chungang* 2, no. 1 (1934): 71–72.

38. See his "Puin ŭi hwa wa naeng" ["Fire" and "cold" in women], *Hanbang ŭihak* 30:11–16.

39. Cho lists some *hanbang* prescriptions effective in addressing bodily weaknesses in his "Puinbyŏng ŭi sŏbyang kwa ch'iryo [Managing and treating *puinbyŏng*]," *Ch'unch'u* (January 1944): 76–81.

40. "Yŏ'ŭi chwadamhoe."

41. Rosetta Sherwood Hall, "A Gynecological Dispensary in Korea," *China Medical Journal* 30, no. 5 (1916): 316–320.

42. Dr. Stewart and Naomi Anderson, "Medical Report of Harris Hospital," *KWC* 17 (1915): 50–53.

43. Pyŏn Ingi, "Puinbyŏng kangjwa 2, woe aegirŭl mot natnŭnga" [*Puinbyŏng* lecture 2, why one cannot have a baby], *Nongmin saenghwal* 12, no. 8 (1940): 26–29.

44. *Tonga ilbo*, May 25, 1928.

45. Yang Hyŏna, "Hoju chedo: Hanguk ŭi singminjisŏnggwa kabujangje ŭi ch'ukto" [The family-headship system: The epitome of Korean coloniality and patriarchy], in *Kyŏnggye ŭi yŏsngtŭl*, ed. Seoul National University Institute for Gender Research (*Yŏsŏng yŏngukso*), 40–78.

46. An example of an article that emphasized proper medical care in childbearing is Chŏn Hŭngsun, "Puinbyŏng e taehaya [About *puinbyŏng*]," *Nongmin saenghwal* 3, no. 6 (June 1931): 36–38. *Nongmin saenghwal* was the journal of a Pyongyang-based association involved in the Christian rural revitalization movement of the late 1920s and early 1930s. Chŏn was a physician at the Christian hospital in Pyongyang.

47. For an analysis of "Underground Village," see Kyeong-Hee Choi, "Impaired Body as Colonial Trope: Kang Kyŏngae's 'Underground Village,'" *Public Culture* 13, no. 3 (2001): 431–458.

48. Hŏ Sin, "Sanbuingwa purimjŭng ch'iryonŭn ŏttŏkke?" *Sin kajŏng* (November 1934): 58–64.

49. Physician critiques of female itinerant healers may be found in articles such as "Yŏ'ŭi chwadamhoe" and "Sanbuingwa chŏnmunŭi ŭi imsin punman sŏpsaeng chwadamhoe" [Roundtable among obstetric-gynecologists on care during pregnancy and delivery], *Chogwang* 3, no. 11 (1937): 156–163. Physicians who participated include Kil Chŏnghui of Hansŏng clinic; Chang Mungyŏng, who had her own practice and contributed many articles on women's health; Pyŏn Sŏkhwa of Severance; Son Ch'ijŏng; Ryu Yŏngjun, medical advisor at Ewha Girls' School; Kim Sŏkhwan of Keijo Imperial University Hospital; Sin P'ilho, former physician at Severance who opened his own practice; Yun T'aegwŏn of the Keijo municipal public hospital; and Hŏ Sin.

50. Yun T'aegwŏn also noted the recovery of fertility after treating a prolapsed uterus in "San puingwaŭi ŭi ilgi" [Journal of an obstetric-gynecologist], *Chogwang* 6, no. 7 (1940): 188–191.

51. "Pyeng Yang Woman's Hospital of Extended Grace," *KWC* 19 (1917): 105–112. While no author is listed, it was likely Rosetta S. Hall, who was stationed there at the time.

52. Mary S. Stewart, MD, and Naomi A. Anderson, Graduate Nurse, "East Gate Medical Work," *KWC* 18 (1916): 60–62.

53. GGK, *Tōkei nenpō*, 1930.

54. Hŏ Sin, "Purimjŭng" [Infertility], *Sin yŏsŏng* 8, no. 1 (1934): 100–103.

55. Mary Cutler, "Woman's Hospital of Extended Grace and Medical Education for Korean Women," *KWC* 20 (1918).

56. For dangers of childbirth in the West, see works such as Judith Leavitt, *Brought to Bed: Childbearing in America, 1750–1950* (New York and Oxford: Oxford University Press, 1986), and Edward Shorter, *Women's Bodies: A Social History of Women's Encounter with Health, Ill-health, and Medicine*, 2nd ed. (New Brunswick, NJ, and London: Transaction Publishers, 1991).

57. Rickets is the softening of bones that results from insufficient absorption of calcium. This condition is often seen in young children, and can lead to fractures and deformities, especially of the pelvic bones of young girls. It is thought to be caused primarily by a deficiency of vitamin D, a necessary vitamin for calcium absorption, or lack of calcium in the diet. While studies in the West indicated that rickets in women as children often led to childbearing difficulties, there is less mention of rickets in and of itself, relative to other factors, as a particular problem for childbearing in popular medical tracts in Korea. The Korean discourse, however, does mention deformities or anomalies as potentially complicating childbearing. In one

case in Pyongyang that received mention in the *Tonga ilbo*, a woman with rickets was subjected to delivery by caesarean at the Pyongyang Provincial Hospital and had her ovaries removed to prevent future pregnancies. See "Kurunŭn imsin pulga" [Rickets makes pregnancy impossible], *Tonga ilbo*, January 31, 1926.

58. "Interview with Dr. PP," *Sanbuingwa ŭisa kusul charyo*.
59. "Yŏ'ŭi chwadamhoe" and "Sanbuingwa chŏnmunŭi ŭi imsin punman sŏpsaeng chwadamhoe." The term used for "midwife" here was usually *nop'a*, literally "elderly woman," who was usually locally known and sought to assist in delivery of children at home. These women were distinguished from *sanp'a*, the common term used to designate younger, educated women trained and licensed in modern midwifery.
60. Yun T'aegwŏn, "Sanbuingwaŭi ŭi ilgi."
61. Theodore Jun Yoo, *It's Madness*, 10.
62. Kim Sŏkhwan, "Sanbuingwaŭi ŭi ilgil," [Journal of an obstetric-gynecologist], *Chogwang* 6, no. 7 (1940): 184–187.
63. "Yŏ'ŭi chwadamhoe."
64. In 1938, they made up about half of the advertised products in the daily newspaper, the *Tonga ilbo*. Shin In Sup and Shin Kie Hyuk, *Advertising in Korea* (Seoul: Communication Books Publications, 2004), 44.
65. See Yi Kkonme, "Ilbanin ŭi hanŭihak insik kwa ŭiyak iyong" [A study on the general public understanding and utilization of traditional Korean medicine in the colonial period]," in *Hanŭihak, singminji rŭl alt'a: singminji sigi hanŭihak ŭi kŭndaehwa yŏngu* [The modernization of Korean traditional medicine during the colonial period], ed. Institute for History of Medicine, Yonsei University (Seoul, Korea: Ak'anet, 2008), 137–154.
66. Ibid., 145. While the example here is of syphilis and not *puinbyŏng*, I include this in the discussion as venereal disease medications often were advertised along with medications specifically addressing *puinbyŏng* or other reproductive system ailments.
67. Susan Burns, "Marketing Health and the Modern Body: Patent Medicine Advertising in Meiji-Taishō Japan," in *Looking Modern: East Asian Visual Culture from Treaty Ports to World War II*, ed. Jennifer Purtle and Hans Thomsen (Chicago: Center for the Art of East Asia, University of Chicago Press, 2009), 179–202.
68. Jin-kyung Park, "Managing 'Dis-ease': Print Media, Medical Images, and Patent Medicine Advertisements in Colonial Korea," *International Journal of Cultural Studies*. First published January 13, 2017.

69. *Chogwang* (July 1941).
70. The version of the advertisement analyzed here is from *Yŏsŏng* 3, no. 1 (1938): 31.
71. *Ch'unch'u* (March 1942). The name evokes the fusion of estrogen and hormone. Other Japanese-patented products that address women-specific ailments marketed and sold in colonial Korea include Wasedon and Chujūto. See analysis of these products in Jin-kyung Park, "Corporeal Colonialism: Medicine, Reproduction, and Race in Colonial Korea" (PhD diss., University of Illinois, Urbana-Champaign, 2008), and Susan Burns, "Marketing Health and the Modern Body."
72. Hong Hyŏn'o, *Hanguk yagŏpsa* [History of Korean pharmacy] (Seoul: Handok yakp'um kongŏp chusik hoesa, 1972), 116. Translations of T'aeyang Chogyŏnghwan and Paekpohwan are taken from So Young Suh, "Korean Medicine Between the Local and the Universal."
73. So Young Suh, "Korean Medicine Between the Local and the Universal," 232.
74. Hong Hyŏn'o, *Hanguk yagŏpsa*, 16.
75. Misinhwan appeared frequently throughout the 1930s and early 1940s. The ads analyzed here appeared in *Chogwang* (August 1936) and *Ch'unch'u* (October 1941).
76. This Misinhwan advertisement is from *Yŏsŏng* 3, no. 8 (1938): 45. Multiple versions of T'aeyangjogyŏnghwan with images of mothers and/or children were advertised throughout the 1910s in the *Maeil sinbo*.
77. A quick survey finds it running from the 1920s into the 1940s in both newspapers and women's journals. A product called Inochi No Haha is sold in Japan today. Interestingly, the contemporary version claims to be a hormonal balancer targeting postmenopausal women.
78. "Mirŭl ilkko 'a-i' rŭl mot natge hanŭn puinbyŏng (chagungbyŏng) ŭi son swi-un chat'aek yobŏp," *Tonga ilbo*, November 19, 1932. The latter articles appear on a one-page spread in *Tonga ilbo*, December 14, 1935. The product was not affordable by many as a one-week supply cost one to two yen, and a three- to four-month supply would cost thirty yen. This was at a time (1931) when the average female worker in Korea earned about thirty sen a day.
79. *Tonga ilbo*, August 13, 1922.
80. "Ch'anggi sain e ŭiun," *Tonga ilbo*, January 25, 1939.
81. Written by Wi Chongch'ŏl, "Miscarriage" was serialized in *Maeil sinbo* from January 14 to 21, 1931. For a longer description of the story, see Sonja Kim, "'Limiting Birth': Birth Control in Colonial Korea (1910–1945)," *EASTS* 2 (2008): 335–359.

82. The fictional physician here hoped for more open approval of birth control in order to materially profit from his practice. *Pyŏlgŏngon* 26 (1930): 40.

83. Sin Tongun, "Hyŏngbŏp kaejŏng kwa kwallyŏn pon nakt'aejoe yŏngu" [A study of abortion from the viewpoint of criminal law reform in Korea], *Hyŏngsa chŏngch'aek yŏngu* [Study of criminal policy] 2, no. 2 (1991): 333–381.

84. On Japanese pronatalist policies, see Helen Hopper, *Katō Shidzue:A Japanese Feminist* (New York: Pearson Education, Inc., 2004); Sabine Frühstück, *Colonizing Sex*; Tiana Norgren, *Abortion Before Birth Control: The Politics of Reproduction in Postwar Japan* (Princeton, NJ: Princeton University Press, 2001); and Sumiko Otsubo, "The Female Body and Eugenic Thought in Meiji Japan," in *Building a Modern Japan: Science, Technology, and Medicine in the Meiji Era and Beyond*, ed. Morris Low (New York: Palgrave Macmillan, 2005), 61–81.

85. Jin-kyung Park, "Corporeal Colonialism."

86. For Japanese medical research on colonized female bodies, see Jin-kyung Park, "Husband Murder as the 'Sickness' of Korea"; "Bodies for Empire: Biopolitics, Reproduction, and Sexual Knowledge in Late Colonial Korea," *Ŭisahak* 23, no. 2 (2014): 203–238; "Picturing Empire and Illness"; "Yellow Men's Burden: East Asian Imperialism, Forensic Medicine, and Conjugality in Colonial Korea," *Acta Koreana* 18, no. 1 (2015): 187–207; and Hong Yanghŭi, "Singminjisigi 'ŭihak' 'chisik' kwa Chosŏn ŭi 'chŏngt'ong': K'udoŭi 'puingwahak'chŏk chungsimŭro" ["Medical knowledge" and "tradition" of colonial Korea: Focused on Kudo's "gynecology"-based knowledge], *Ŭisahak* 22, no. 2 (2013): 579–616.

87. *Tonga ilbo*, August 16–22, 1921.

88. The discourse on the "population problem" in colonial Korea covered a broad array of issues from food shortages, overpopulation, rural impoverishment, urban migrations, and population mobilizations, including the encouragement of Koreans to resettle in Manchuria or other parts of the Japanese empire.

89. Karen Lee Callahan, "Dangerous Devices, Mysterious Times: Men, Women, and Birth Control in Early Twentieth-Century Japan" (PhD diss., University of California, Berkeley, 2004).

90. How the X-ray was used as a sterilization method was not clarified in these articles. One example of detailed instructions on the rhythm method is "Sana chehan ŭi sae pogŭm, yak ssŭji annŭn p'iimbŏp, puinegenŭn purim il i itda. Chugi kŭmyokŭro p'iim ikanŭng" [New blessing in "limiting

birth," contraceptive method that does not use drugs, which can bring infertility to women. Contraception is possible with "periodic abstinence"], *Sin kajŏng* 1, no. 6 (1933): 142–145.

91. Koreans called the rhythm method, "periodic abstinence" or the Ogino method, named after the Japanese physician who popularized the method.

92. An T'aeyun, *Singminji chŏngch'i wa mosŏng*.

93. Pak Hojin, "Sanmo poho wa injong kaeryang pangmyŏn" [Protecting maternity and improving the race], *Samch'ŏlli* no. 5 (1930).

94. "Kyŏrhon chŏn kwa kyŏrhon hu [Before and after marriage]," *Tonggwang* 39 (1932): 63–64.

95. "An interview with Na Hyesŏk, 'U'ae kyŏrhon, sihŏm kyŏrhon'" [Companionate marriage, trial marriage], *Samch'ŏlli* 6 (1930): 53–54, part of roundtable discussion, "Sin yangsŏng todŏk ŭi chech'ang" [Proposal for new morality for both sexes].

96. Yun Sŏngsang, "Sana chehan ŭi chŏlgyu: sŏnjŏn kwa sirhaeng ŭi p'ilyo" [An urgent call for birth control: Need for awareness and practice], *Samch'ŏlli* 5 (1930): 53–57. Yun also was a graduate of the colonial government's Teacher Training School.

97. This observation was also made by Theodore Jun Yoo and So Hyŏnsuk. Theodore Jun Yoo, "The 'New Woman' and the Politics of Love, Marriage and Divorce in Colonial Korea," *Gender & History* 17, no. 2 (2005): 295–324, and So Hyŏnsuk, "Ilche sigi ch'ulsan chehan tamnon yŏngu" [Study of the birth control discourse in colonial Korea], *Yŏksa wa hyŏnsil* 38 (2000): 221–253.

98. "Myŏngnyu puin kwa sana chehan" [Famous women and birth control], *Samch'olli* 8 (1930): 50–54.

99. Pae Sŏngnyong, "Sana chehan ŭi hyŏnsilsŏng, Chosŏn ŭi kyŏngjae chŏngse wa saenghwal hyŏngt'ae e kamhaya" [Reality of limiting birth, state of Chosŏn's economy and everyday life], *Samch'ŏlli*, no. 5 (1930): 30–32.

100. Concern over physical harm caused by contraceptive devices culminated in the 1930 legislation in Japan abolishing intrauterine contraceptive devices. Callahan, "Dangerous Devices, Mysterious Times."

101. "Sana chojŏlŭl haeya hana? Modudŭl haeyahandamnida" [Should you practice birth control? Everyone should], *Yŏsŏng* 1, no. 1 (1936): 16–17.

102. Pak Hwich'un, "Sahoechŏk kyonjiesŏ sana chehand ŭi hyŏnsiljŏk pip'an" [Realistic critique of birth limitation from a social perspective], *Sil saeng-hwal* 5, no. 6 (1934): 1–3.

103. This logic was also wielded by opponents of birth control who believed birth control would prevent the birth of potential heroes and leaders. Pak Hwich'un, "Sahoechŏk kyonjiesŏ sana chehan ŭi hyŏnsiljŏk pip'an."

104. At the forefront of the eugenics movement, he wrote prolifically on the topic. Some titles include, "Birth Control Seen from the Perspective of Eugenics," "A Few Words on the Problem of Marriage," *Chosŏn ilbo*, September 27–October 1, 1933. "What Is the Eugenics Movement?" *Chunggang* (November 1933); and "Treatise on Eugenic Birth Control," *Sin yŏsŏng* 7, no. 8 (1933): 76–79.

105. Yun Ch'iho was a prominent Protestant literary figure and nationalist leader in colonial Korea. Moderate leftist Yŏ Ŭnhyŏng was an organizer of the Korea Provisional Government in Shanghai in the 1920s and emerged postliberation as a major contender to lead the newly independent Korean nation before his untimely assassination in 1947. Kim Hwallan (Helen Kim), a champion of female education, was the first Korean president of Ewha Womans University. Among the Association's initial eighty-five members, twenty-five graduated from medical school. Christian leaders formed a large part of the membership as well. In its by-laws, the Association states that it "aims to promote the happiness of society by improving the physiques and minds of future descendants through eugenic means." This was to be done by conducting surveys, researching eugenic theory and application, spreading eugenic knowledge among the populace, publishing a journal, and offering consultation on infant welfare and eugenic marriage. The organization was active until 1937, during which time it sponsored lectures, held roundtable discussions, and published three issues of its journal *Usaeng*.

106. "Ilbon yŏgong ŭi purimjŭng, Chosŏn yŏjagongtŭlŭn kwayŏn ŏttŏhanga?" [Infertility in Japanese women factory workers. What about in Korea?], *Tonga ilbo*, March 19, 1924.

107. Pyŏn Sŏkhwa, "Chigŏp yŏsŏng ŭi pogŏn e taehaŏ" [Health of working women], *Sin kajŏng* (February 1935): 104–109.

108. Pyŏn Ingi, "Puinbyŏng kangjwa 1 [*Puinbyŏng* lecture 1]," *Nongmin saenghwal* 12, no. 7 (1940): 29–31.

109. "Naega manil yŏsŏn undonggamyŏn?" *Sin kajŏng* (April 1933).

110. "Segye kakkuk ŭi pogŏn sisŏl" [Health facilities in other countries], *Sin tonga* (March 1933): 6–9.

111. Yi Sŏngŭn, "T'aegyo ŭi kwahakchŏk ŭmmi" [Scientific examination of prenatal education], *Sin tonga* (January 1931): 5–7.

112. Dikötter, *Sex, Culture, and Modernity in China*, 42–44.

113. The *kisaeng* journal *Chang Han* included a section on gynecological health in each of the extant issues I examined. Issues discussed included women's menstrual cycle and venereal diseases such as syphilis and gonorrhea. For more on this journal, see Ruth Barraclough, "The Courtesan's Journal: Kisaeng and the Sex Labour Market in Colonial Korea," *Intersections: Gender and Sexuality in Asia and the Pacific* 29 (2012): 1–9.

EPILOGUE

1. Hŏ explained her visions for Korea's first maternity clinic a few years before it opened. Hŏ Yŏngsuk, "Tonggyŏng e ŏtjae watdŭngo, sanwŏn e taehan naŭi kudo" [Returning from Tokyo, my thoughts on maternity clinics], *Samch'ŏlli* 8, no. 4 (1936): 111–113. The opening of the clinic was reported in "Yŏng'a ŭi agwŏn Hŏ Yŏngsuk sanwŏn" [An infant clinic, Hŏ Yŏngsuk Maternity Clinic], *Samch'ŏlli* 10, no. 8 (1938): 160–161.
2. "Ch'ogi saŏp ŭro 9 wŏl put'ŏ kangsŭphoe" [Training institute as first project, starting in September], *Tonga ilbo*, May 21, 1928.
3. "Naega pon na, myŏngsa ŭi cha'a'gwan," *Pyŏlgŏngon* 29 (1930): 57.
4. Kwŏn Sangja, "Kyŏngsŏng myŏnginmul [sŭmyŏn] rok," *Pyŏlgŏngon* 34 (1930): 108.
5. Japan established the puppet government of Manchukuo in 1932 and invaded China in 1937, setting off the second Sino-Japanese War. The East Asian Co-Prosperity Sphere was established in 1940 as Japan moved to incorporate Southeast and East Asia into its empire. This aggression exacerbated tensions between Japan and the United States, which culminated in the attack on Pearl Harbor and U.S. entry into World War II.
6. Takashi Fujitani, "Right to Kill, Right to Make Live: Koreans as Japanese and Japanese as Americans During WWII," *Representations* 99 (2007): 15.
7. Ibid., 21.
8. Kil Chŏnghŭi, *Na ŭi chasŏjŏn*, 38.
9. According to Karen Lee Callahan, Ishimoto Shizue's arrest was part of a general repression of left-wing activism, under which label birth control advocacy now belonged. Ishimoto was released ten days after her arrest and compelled to close her birth control clinics. Callahan, "Dangerous Devices, Mysterious Times."
10. An T'aeyun, *Singmin chŏngch'i wa mosŏng*, 128.

11. The Bureau also sought to introduce countermeasures against tuberculosis and venereal diseases, which were blamed for the low-level quality of military recruits.
12. An T'aeyun, *Singmin chŏngch'i wa mosŏng*, 129.
13. Pronatalist policies, however, contradicted other policies enacted by the colonial government, such as the military sexual slavery system, which distributed condoms (while restricting their circulation among the general population) through the military to its various comfort women stations as well as performing abortions on pregnant comfort women. Kang Chŏngsuk, "Ilbongun 'Wianbu' chejo wa kiŏp ŭi yŏkhal—satk'u (k'ondom) rŭl chungsimŭro" [The Japanese military "comfort woman" system and role of enterprises—focus on the condom], *Yŏksa pip'yŏng* 60 (2002): 270–288.
14. Frühstück, *Colonizing Sex*, 166.
15. Compulsory sterilization was barely enforced, however, reflecting the imperial government's pronatalist leanings. Researchers have unearthed that during the war in Japan, only a total of 454 persons were sterilized in accordance with the law. An T'aeyun, "Ilcheha mosŏng," 81.
16. Callahan, "Dangerous Devices, Mysterious Times," 191–192.
17. In Korea, young persons were encouraged to visit marriage consultation centers and receive examination for potential genetic conditions or presence of sexually transmitted disease.
18. Sin Yŏngjŏn, "Singminji Chosŏn esŏ usaeng undong ŭi chŏngae wa sŏnggyŏk: 1930 nyŏndae 'Usaeng' ŭl chungsimŭro" [The characteristics of Korea's eugenic movement in the colonial period represented in the bulletin *Usaeng*], *Ŭisahak* 15, no. 2 (2006): 133–155.
19. Eunjung Kim, *Curative Violence: Rehabilitating Disability, Gender, and Sexuality in Modern Korea* (Durham, NC: Duke University Press, 2017), 64.
20. "Interview with Dr. PP," *Sanbuingwa kusul charyo*.
21. This is not to say that it is popularly accepted today but that state public health programs and the medical field in general operate on such logic.
22. For example, fertility treatment in medical tourism and biotechnological research is heavily promoted by the state; public service announcements and various incentives at local borough and private levels encourage families to have more children; and maternity clinics (*sanhu choriwŏn*) that focus on the postpartum care of mothers have emerged as a lucrative market. For more on South Korea's 1960s family planning campaigns and their engagement with international health organizations and domestic

medical health administration, see John DiMoia "알맞게 낳아서 훌륭하게 기르자! (Let's Have the Proper Number of Children and Raise Them Well): Family Planning and Nation-Building in South Korea, 1961–1968," *EASTS* 2, no. 3 (2008): 361–379.

23. The distribution of the organization's members in the medical specialties of pediatrics and obstetrics-gynecology were even at 22.8 percent each (totaling 45.6 percent of the membership). Of the remaining 20 specialties represented, internal medicine followed with less than 10 percent. Hanguk yŏja ŭisahoe, *Hanguk yŏja ŭisa 90 nyŏn*, 142–143.

24. According to one report, South Korea touts the lowest fertility rate among Organisation for Economic Co-operation and Development (OECD) member countries in the world. "Already OECD Lowest, South Korea's Birthrate Getting Worse," *The Hankyoreh*, August 28, 2016, http://english.hani.co.kr/arti/english_edition/e_national/758664.html, accessed March 11, 2017.

BIBLIOGRAPHY

NEWSPAPERS AND JOURNALS

Bulletin of the Nurses' Association of Korea—Chosŏn kanhobu hoebo
Chang Han
Cheguk sinmun
The China Medical Journal
Chogwang
Chosŏn ilbo
Chosŏn ŭibo
Ch'unch'u
Chungang
Hanbang ŭihak
Honam hakpo
Hwangsŏng sinmun
Hyŏndae puin
Kidok sinmun
The Korea Mission Field
Kyo'u hoeji (Kyŏngsŏng yŏja ŭihak kangsŭpso)
Maeil sinbo
Nongmin saenghwal
Pyŏlgŏngon
Samch'ŏlli
Sil saenghwal
Sin kajŏng
Sin yŏja
Sin yŏsŏng

Sŏbuk hakhoe wŏlbo
Taehan hŭnghakpo
Tonga ilbo
Tonggwang
Tongnip sinmun
Tongsŏ ŭihak
Tongsŏ ŭihak yŏnguhoe wŏlbo
Yŏjagye
Yŏsŏng

OTHER SOURCES

Allen, Horace. *Allen ŭi ilgi* [Horace Allen's diary], translated by Kim Won-jo. Seoul: Dankook University Press, 1991.

An Chonghwa, trans. *Ch'odŭng saengni wisaenghak taeyo* [An elementary outline on physiology and hygiene]. Hansŏng (Seoul): Kwangdŏk sŏgwan, 1909.

———, trans. *Ch'odŭng yulli kyogwasŏ* [Elementary ethics textbook] (1907). Reprinted in *Hanguk kaehwagi kyogwasŏ ch'ongsŏ* 10. Seoul: Asea munhwasa, 1977.

An Sanggyŏng. "Chosŏn sidae ŭi ŭinyŏ chedo e kwanhan yŏngu" [A study on the *ŭinyŏ* system in the Chosŏn dynasty]. PhD diss., Kyŏngsan University, 2000.

An T'aeyun. *Singminji chŏngch'i wa mosŏng: ch'ongdongwŏn ch'eje wa mosŏng ŭi hyŏnsil* [The politics of motherhood in colonial Korea]. P'aju, South Korea: Hanguk haksul chŏngbo, 2006.

Apple, Rima D. "Constructing Mothers: Scientific Mothering in the Nineteenth and Twentieth Centuries." *Social History of Medicine* 8, no. 2 (1995): 161–178.

Baker, Donald. "Oriental Medicine in Korea." In *Medicine Across Cultures: History and Practice of Medicine in Non-Western Cultures*, edited by H. Selin, 133–153. Dordrecht, The Netherlands: Kluwer Academic Publishers, 2003.

Barraclough, Ruth. "The Courtesan's Journal: Kisaeng and the Sex Labour Market in Colonial Korea." *Intersections: Gender and Sexuality in Asia and the Pacific* 29 (2012): 1–9.

Bart, Richard Quain, ed. *A Dictionary of Medicine: Including General Pathology, General Therapeutics, Hygiene, and the Diseases of Women and Children*. New York: D. Appleton and Company, 1895.

Burns, Susan. "Marketing Health and the Modern Body: Patent Medicine Advertising in Meiji-Taishō Japan." In *Looking Modern: East Asian Visual Culture from Treaty Ports to World War II*, edited by Jennifer Purtle and Hans Thomsen, 179–202. Chicago: Center for the Art of East Asia, University of Chicago Press, 2009.

Callahan, Karen Lee. "Dangerous Devices, Mysterious Times: Men, Women, and Birth Control in Early Twentieth-Century Japan." PhD diss., University of California, Berkeley, 2004.

Caprio, Mark. "Abuse of Modernity: Japanese Biological Determinism and Identity Management in Colonial Korea." *Cross-Currents: East Asian History and Culture Review* 10 (2014). https://cross-currents.berkeley.edu/e-journal/issue-10

Caprio, Mark E. *Japanese Assimilation Policies in Colonial Korea, 1910–1945*. Seattle: University of Washington Press, 2009.

Chang Chiyŏn. *Yŏja tokpon* (1908), edited and translated by Mun Hyeyun. Kwangmyŏng, South Korea: Kyŏngjin, 2012.

Cho, Byong-Hee. "The State and Physicians in South Korea, 1910–1985: An Analysis of Professionalization." PhD diss., University of Wisconsin–Madison, 1988.

Cho Kyŏngwŏn. "Taehan cheguk mal yŏhaksaeng kyogwasŏ e nat'anan yŏsŏng kyoyuk ron ŭi t'ŭksŏng kwa hangye" [A content analysis of textbooks for female students in the end of the Taehan empire period]. *Kyoyuk kwahak yŏngu* 30 (1999): 163–187.

Ch'oe Ŭngyŏng (Choi, Eun-Kyung). "Ilche kangjŏmgi Chosŏn yŏja ŭisadŭl ŭi hwaltong—Tokyo yŏja ŭihakkyo chorŏp 4 inŭl chungsimŭro" [The activities of women physicians in colonial Korea—focusing on four graduates of Tokyo Women's Medical College]. *Cogito* 80 (2016): 287–316.

Chohŏn wanghu Han ssi and Song Siyŏl. *Sinwanyŏk Naehun, Kyenyŏsŏ* [New translation of *Naehun* and *Kyenyŏsŏ*], translated by Kim Chonggwŏn. Seoul: Myŏngmundang, 1987.

Choi, Hyaeweol. *Gender and Mission Encounters in Korea: New Women, Old Ways*. Berkeley: University of California Press, 2009.

———. "The Missionary Home as a Pulpit: Domestic Paradoxes in Early Twentieth-Century Korea." In *Divine Domesticities: Christian Paradoxes in Asia and the Pacific*, edited by Margaret Jolly and Hyaeweol Choi, 29–55. Canberra: Australian National University Press, 2014.

———. "'Wise Mother, Good Wife': A Transcultural Discursive Construct in Modern Korea." *The Journal of Korean Studies* 14, no. 1 (2009): 1–34.

Choi, Kyeong-Hee. "Impaired Body as Colonial Trope: Kang Kyŏngae's 'Underground Village.'" *Public Culture* 13, no. 3 (2001): 431–458.

Chŏn Migyŏng. "1900–1910 nyŏndae kajŏng kyogwasŏ e kwanhan yŏngu: Hyŏn Kongnyŏm parhaeng *Hanmun kajŏnghak, Sinp'yŏn kajŏnghak, Sinjŏng kajŏnghak ŭl chungsimŭro*" [A study of home economics textbooks, 1900– 1910: An analysis of *Hanmun kajŏnghak, Sinp'yŏn kajŏnghak,* and *Sinjŏng kajŏnghak* published by Hyŏn Kongnyŏm]. *Hanguk kajŏngkwa kyoyukhak hoeji* 17, no. 1 (2005): 131–151.

———. "1920–30 nyŏndae hyŏnmo yangch'ŏ e kwanhan yŏngu: hyŏnmo yanchŏ ŭi tu ŏlgul, toe'ŏyaman hanŭn 'hyŏnmo' toego sip'ŭn 'yangchŏ'" [Discourse on "Wise Mother and Good Wife" in the 1920s–1930s: Women's ambivalence about the roles of Wise Mother and Good Wife]. *Hanguk kajŏng kwallihak hoeji* 22, no. 2 (2004): 75–93.

———. "Singminji sidae 'Kasa kyogwasŏ' e kwanhan yŏngu: 1930 nyŏndaerŭl chungsimŭro" [Analysis of household textbooks for middle high school in colonial age]. *Hanguk kajŏnggwa kyoyukhak hoeji* 16, no. 3 (2004): 1–25.

Chŏng Chihun. "Ilche sidae hanŭi haksul chapchi yŏngu" [Research on academic journals of oriental medicine in the era of Japanese imperialism]. *Hanguk ŭisahak hoeji* 14, no. 2 (2001): 173–188.

Chŏng Chunyŏng, "Singminji ŭihak kyoyuk kwa hegemŏni kyŏngjaeng: Kyŏngsŏng chedae ŭihakpu ŭi sŏllip kwajŏng kwa chedojŏk t'ŭkjingŭl chungsimŭro" [Medical education and competition for hegemony in colonial Korea: Establishment and characteristic of Keijō Imperial University Medical Department]. *Sahoe wa hyŏnsil* 85 (2010): 197–237.

Chōsen sōtokofu. *Chōsen jinkō genshō* [Korea's population issue]. Keijō (Seoul), 1926.

———. *Chōsen no jinkō no mondai* [Korea's population problem]. Keijō (Seoul), 1935.

———. Chōsen sōtokofu keimu sōkanfu, *Chōsen eisei hōkishū* [Compilation of Chosŏn hygiene regulations]. Keijō (Seoul), 1917.

———. *Chōsen sōtokofu tōkei nenpō* [Annual statistics report of the Government-General of Korea]. Keijō (Seoul), 1910–1942.

Chosŏn wangjo sillok [Annals of the Chosŏn dynasty]. http://sillok .history.go.kr/main/main.do

Cooter, Roger, ed. *In the Name of the Child: Health and Welfare, 1880–1940.* London and New York: Routledge, 1992.

Deuchler, Martina. *Confucian Transformation of Korea: A Study of Society and Ideology.* Cambridge, MA: Council on East Asian Studies and Harvard University Press, 1992.

———. "Propagating Female Virtues in Chosŏn Korea." In *Women and Confucian Cultures in Premodern China, Korea, and Japan,* edited by Dorothy

Ko, JaHyun Haboush, and Joan Piggott, 142–169. Berkeley, Los Angeles, and London: University of California Press, 2003.

Dikötter, Frank. *Sex, Culture, and Modernity in China: Medical Science and the Construction of Sexual Identities in the Early Republican Period.* Honolulu: University of Hawai'i Press, 1995.

DiMoia, John. *Reconstructing Bodies: Biomedicine, Health, and Nation-Building in South Korea Since 1945.* Redwood City, CA: Stanford University Press, 2013.

———. "알맞게 낳아서 훌륭하게 기르자! (Let's Have the Proper Number of Children and Raise Them Well!): Family Planning and Nation-Building in South Korea, 1961–1968." *East Asian Science, Technology, and Society: An International Journal* [EASTS] 2 (2008): 361–379.

Dittrich, Klaus. "The Beginnings of Modern Education in Korea, 1883–1910." *Paedagogica Histories* 50, no. 3 (2014): 265–284.

Duncan, John. "The *Naehun* and the Politics of Gender in Fifteenth-Century Korea." In *Creating Women of Korea: The Fifteenth through the Twentieth Centuries*, edited by Young-Key Kim-Renaud, 26–57. Armonk, NY: M. E. Sharpe, 2004.

Ewha kajŏnghak 50 nyŏnsa [Fifty-year history of home economics at Ewha]. Seoul: Ihwa yŏja taehak kajŏng taehak, 1979.

Fifty Years of Light. Seoul: Woman's Foreign Missionary Society of the Methodist Episcopal Church, 1938.

Frühstück, Sabine. *Colonizing Sex: Sexology and Social Control in Modern Japan.* Berkeley and Los Angeles: University of California Press, 2003.

Fujitani, Takashi. "Right to Kill, Right to Make Live: Koreans as Japanese and Japanese as Americans During WWII." *Representations* 99 (Summer 2007): 13–39.

Furth, Charlotte. *A Flourishing Yin: Gender in China's Medical History, 960–1665.* Berkeley and Los Angeles: University of California Press, 1999.

Government General of Chosen. *Manual of Education in Chosen (1920)*, Appendix, 13. Reprinted in *Singminji Chosŏn kyoyuk chŏngch'aek saryo chipsŏng* [Sources on educational policy in colonial Korea], vol. 2. Seoul: Taehaksŏwŏn, 1990.

Hall, Sherwood. *With Stethoscope in Asia.* McLean, VA: MCL Associates, 1978.

Hanguk kŭndae hakkyo kyoyuk 100 nyŏnsa yŏngu [One hundred years of the history of education in Korean modern schools], vols. 1–2. Seoul: Hanguk kyoyuk kaebarwŏn, 1994 and 1997.

Hanguk yŏja ŭisahoe. *Hanguk yŏja ŭisa 90 nyŏn* [Ninety years of female physicians in Korea]. Seoul: Ŭihak ch'ulpansa, 1986.

Hanŭihak ŭi pip'an kwa haesŏl. Seoul: Sonamu, 1997.

Harrell, Paula. "The Meiji 'New Woman' and China." In *Late Qing China and Meiji Japan: Political and Cultural Aspects,* edited by Joshua A. Fogel, 109–150. Norwalk, CT: EastBridge, 2004.

Häußler, Sonja. "Kyubang Kasa: Women's Writings from the Late Chosŏn." In *Creative Women of Korea,* edited by Young-Key Kim-Renaud, 142–162.

Henry, Todd. *Assimilating Seoul: Japanese Rule and the Politics of Public Space in Colonial Korea, 1910–1945.* Berkeley and Los Angeles: University of California Press, 2014.

———. "Sanitizing Empire: Articulations of Korean Otherness and the Construction of Early Colonial Seoul, 1905–1919." *Journal of Asian Studies* 64, no. 3 (2005): 639–675.

Hŏ Chaeyŏng et al., ed. and trans. *Kŭndae susin kyogwasŏ* [Modern moral textbooks]. Seoul: Somyŏng ch'ulp'an, 2011.

Hŏ Chun and the *Tongŭi pogam* kuḡyŏk wiwŏnhoe [Committee on the vernacular translation of the *Tongŭi pogam*], *Tongŭi pogam.* Seoul: P'ungnyŏnsa, 1966. (Original work published 1613.)

Hocking, William Ernest. *Re-thinking Missions: A Laymen's Inquiry after One Hundred Years.* New York and London: Harper and Brothers Publishers, 1926.

Hong Hyŏn'o. *Hanguk yagŏpsa* [History of Korean pharmacy]. Seoul: Handok yakp'um kongŏp chusik hoesa, 1972.

Hong Yanghŭi. "Singminjisigi 'ŭihak' 'chisik' kwa Chosŏn ŭi 'chŏngt'ong': K'udoŭi 'puingwahak'chŏk chungsimŭro" ["Medical knowledge" and "tradition" of colonial Korea: Focused on Kudo's "gynecology"-based knowledge]. *Ŭisahak* 22, no. 2 (2013): 579–616.

Hopper, Helen. *Katō Shidzue: A Japanese Feminist.* New York: Pearson Education, Inc., 2004.

Huber, Mary Taylor, and Nancy C. Lutkehaus. "Introduction: Gendered Missions at Home and Abroad." In *Gendered Missions: Women and Men in Missionary Discourse and Practice,* edited by Huber and Lutkehaus, 1–38. Ann Arbor: University of Michigan Press, 1999.

Hwang, Kyung Moon. *Beyond Birth: Social Status in the Emergence of Modern Korea.* Cambridge, MA: Harvard University Asia Center, 2004.

———. *Rationalizing Korea: The Rise of the Modern State, 1894–1945.* Oakland: University of California Press, 2016.

Hwang Misuk. "Sŏngyosa Maren Bordingŭi Kongju, Taejŏn chiyŏk yu'a pokchi wa u'yu kŭpsikso saŏp" [Infant welfare and milk feeding projects of missionary Maren Bording in Kongju and Taejon]. *Hanguk kidokkyo wa yŏksa* 34 (2011): 165–190.

Hyŏn Kongnyŏm, trans. *(Hanmun) Kajŏnghak* [Household management in classical Chinese]. Keijō (Seoul), 1907.

———, trans. *(Sinjŏng) Kajŏnghak* [Household management, newly revised]. Keijō (Seoul), 1913.

———, trans. *(Sinp'yŏn) Kajŏnghak* [Household management, new edition]. Keijō (Seoul), 1907.

Im Chŏngbin. "Kaehwagi Hanguk kajŏng saenghwal: *Maeil sinbo* sasŏl ŭl chungsimŭro" [Korean family life in the early 20th century: Editorials of *Maeil sinbo*]. *Hanguk kajok chawŏn kyŏngyŏnghak hoeji* 3, no. 1 (1999): 1–10.

Johnson, Linda L. "Meiji Women's Educators as Public Intellectuals: Shimoda Utako and Tsuda Umeko." *U.S.-Japan Women's Journal* 44 (2014): 67–92.

Kajŏng kwahak taehak 70 nyŏnsa [Seventy-year history of domestic science college]. Seoul: Ingan saenghwal hwangyŏng yŏnguso, 1999.

Kang Chŏngsuk. "Ilbongun 'Wianbu' chejo wa kiŏp ŭi yŏkhal—satk'u (k'ondom) rŭl chungsimŭro" [The Japanese military 'comfort woman' system and role of enterprises—focus on the condom]. *Yŏksa pip'yŏng* 60 (2002): 270–288.

Kang Myŏngsuk. "Ilche sidae pot'ong hakkyo 'chigŏp' kyogwa ŭi toip kwa kŭ sŏnggyŏk" ["Vocational" subject in normal school during Japanese colonial period]. *Kyoyuk sahak yŏngu* [Study of history of education] 21, no. 2 (2011): 1–33.

———. *Sarip hakkyo ŭi kiwŏn: Ilche ch'ogi hakkyo sŏllip kwa chiyŏk sahoe* [Origins of private schools: Establishment of schools and local society in early colonial Korea]. Seoul: Hagi sisŭp, 2015.

Kang Tŏkhŭi. "Ku Hanmal kaehwagi put'ŏ 8.15 Kwangbok kkaji ŭi kajŏnggwa kyoyuk e kwanhan yŏngu" [Home economics education from late nineteenth century to 1945]. PhD diss., Hanyang University, 1993.

Ki Ch'angdŏk (Kee Chang Duk). *Hanguk kŭndae ŭihak kyoyuksa* [A history of modern medical education in Korea]. Seoul: Academia, 1995.

———. "Kaehwagi ŭi tongŭi wa tongŭihak kangsŭpso" [Oriental medical doctors and the Oriental Medical Training Institute during the Enlightenment period]. *Ŭisahak* 2, no. 2 (1993): 178–196.

———. "Kyŏngsŏng cheguk taehakkyo ŭihakpu" [Medical department of Keijō Imperial University]. *Ŭisahak* 1, no. 1 (1992): 64–82.

———. "Sarip yŏja ŭihak kyoyuk" [The early history of private education of Western medicine for women]. *Ŭisahak* 1, no. 2 (1993): 85–97.

Kil Chŏnghŭi. *Na ŭi chasŏjŏn* [My memoirs]. Seoul: Samho ch'ulp'ansa, 1981.

Kim Chŏnghwa and Yi Kyŏngwŏn. "Ilche singminji chibae wa Chosŏn yangŭi ŭi sahoejŏk sŏnggyŏk" [Japanese rule and social characteristics of physicians of Western medicine in colonial Korea]. *Sahoe wa yŏksa* 70 (2006): 33–65.

Kim Dong-no, John B. Duncan, and Kim Do-hyung, eds. *Reform and Modernity in the Taehan Empire*. Seoul: Jimoondang, 2006.

Kim, Eunjung. *Curative Violence: Rehabilitating Disability, Gender, and Sexuality in Modern Korea*. Durham, NC: Duke University Press, 2017.

Kim Ho. "18 segi huban kŏgyŏng sajok ŭi wisaeng kwa ŭiryo" [Health and medicine of capital-based elite families during the late 18th century]. *Sŏul hak yŏngu* 11 (1998): 113–144.

———. *Hŏ Chun ŭi* Tongŭi pogam *yŏngu* [Study of Hŏ Chun's *Tongŭi pogam*]. Seoul: Ilchisa, 2000.

Kim, Hoi-eun. *Doctors of Empire: Medical and Cultural Encounters between Imperial Germany and Meiji Japan*. Toronto: University of Toronto Press, 2014.

Kim Hyegyŏng. "Kasa nodong tamnon kwa Hanguk kŭndae kajok: 1920–30 nyŏndae rŭl chungsimŭro" [Discourse on housekeeping and Korean modern family of the 1920s and 1930s]. *Hanguk yŏsŏnghak* 15, no. 1 (1999): 153–184.

———. "'Ŏrinigi' ŭi hyŏngsŏng kwa 'mosŏng' ŭi chegusŏng" [The emergence of "childhood" and recomposition of motherhood]. In *Kyŏnggye ŭi yŏsngtŭl: Hanguk kŭndae yŏsŏngsa* [Women on the border: History of women in modern Korea], edited by Seoul National University Institute for Gender Research (*Yŏsŏng yŏngukso*), 79–107. Seoul: Hanul Academy, 2013.

———. *Singminjiha kŭndae kajok ŭi hyŏngsŏng chendŏ* [The formation of the modern family and gender during the colonial period]. Seoul: Ch'angbi Publications, 2006.

Kim, Jisoo M. *Emotions of Justice: Gender, Status, and Legal Performance in Chosŏn Korea*. Seattle: University of Washington Press, 2016.

———. "From Jealousy to Violence: Marriage, Family, and Confucian Patriarchy in Fifteenth-Century Korea." *Acta Koreana* 20, no. 1 (2017): 91–110.

Kim Kŭnbae. *Hanguk kŭndae kwahak kisul illyŏk ŭi ch'ulhyŏn* [The emergence of Korean modern science-technical manpower]. Seoul: Munhak kwa chisŏngsa, 2005.

Kim Kyŏngnam. "Kŭndae kyemonggi kajŏnghak yŏksul choryorŭl t'onghae pon chisik suyong yangsik" [Accommodation of knowledge as seen through the translated compilations on *kajŏnghak* in the modern enlightenment period]. *Inmun kwahak yŏngu* 46 (2015): 5–28.

Kim Minjae. "Kŭndae susin kyogwasŏ t'amsaekk ŭl t'onghan chŏnt'ong kyoyuk kwa hyŏndae todŏkkwa kyoyuk ŭi yŏngyŏl" [Looking at traditional education and contemporary ethics education through *susin* textbooks]. In *Kŭndae hakpu p'yŏnch'an susinsŏ* [*Susin* textbooks published by the modern board of education], edited by Pak Pyŏnggi and Kim Minjae, 212–222. Seoul: Somyŏng, 2012.

Kim Miŭn. "Chosŏn sidae ŭinyŏ chedo e kwanhan koch'al" [Study of Chosŏn period *ŭinyŏ* system]. MA thesis, Kyŏngsŏng University, 2004.

Kim Miyŏng. "Ilche ha *Chosŏn ilbo* ŭi *Kajŏng puin ran yŏngu*" [A study of the *Women's Column* in *Chosŏn ilbo* in colonial Korea]. *Hanguk hyŏndaehak yŏngu* 16 (2004): 221–278.

Kim Ŏnsun. "Kaehwagi yŏsŏng kyoyuk e naejaechŏk yŏsŏnggwan" [Perspectives of women in the education of women in the period of Enlightenment]. *P'eminijŭm yŏngu* 10, no. 2 (2010): 35–87.

Kim Puja. *Hakkyo pak ŭi Chosŏn yŏsŏngtŭl* [Korean women outside of school], translated by Cho Kyŏnghŭi and Kim Uja. Seoul: Ilchogak, 2005.

Kim Sangdŏk. "Yŏja ŭihak kangsŭpso, 1928 nyŏn eŏ 1938 kkaji" [The woman's medical training institute, 1928–1938]. *Ŭisahak* 2, no. 1 (1993): 80–84.

Kim, Sonja. "'Limiting Birth': Birth Control in Colonial Korea." *EASTS* 2, no. 3 (2008): 335–359.

———. "Missionaries and 'A Better Baby Movement' in Colonial Korea." In *Divine Domesticities*, edited by Margaret Jolly and Hyaeweol Choi, 57–83.

———. "The Search for Health: Translating *Wisaeng* and Medicine during the Taehan Empire." In *Reform and Modernity in the Taehan Empire*, edited by Kim et al., 299–341.

Kim Sujin. *Sin yŏsŏng, kŭndae ŭi kwa'ing: singminji Chosŏn ŭi sin yŏsŏng tamnon kwa chendŏ chŏngch'i, 1920–1934* [Excess of the modern: The new woman in colonial Korea]. Seoul: Somyŏng ch'ulp'an, 2009.

Kim Sunjŏn et al. *Cheguk ŭi singminji susin: Chosŏn ch'ongdokpu p'yŏnch'an Susinsŏ yŏngu* [Colonial ethics in the empire: Study of ethics textbooks published by the GGK]. Seoul: JENC, 2009.

———. *Chosŏn ch'ongdokpu ch'odŭng hakkyo susinso* [GGK's elementary school ethics textbooks], vols. 1–2. Seoul: JENC, 2006.

Kim Sunjŏn and Chang Migyŏng. "Chosŏn ch'ongdokpu palgan 'Yŏja kodŭng pot'ong hakkyo susinsŏ' ŭi yŏsŏngsang" [Ideal woman reflected in ethics textbook for Girls' Normal High School published by the Government-General in Korea]. *Ilbonhak yŏnguji* 21 (2007): 155–175.

Kim, Suyun. "Racialization and Colonial Space: Intermarriage in Yi Hyosŏk's Works." *Journal of Korean Studies* 18, no. 1 (2013): 29–59.

Kim Tujong. *Hanguk ŭihaksa chŏn* [History of Korean medicine]. Seoul: T'amgudang, 1966.

Kim, Yung-sik. "Specialized Knowledge in Traditional East Asian Contexts." *EASTS* 4, no. 2 (2010): 179–183.

Klaus, Alisa. *Every Child a Lion: The Origins of Maternal and Infant Health Policy in the US and France, 1890–1920*. Ithaca, NY, and London: Cornell University Press, 1993.

Ko Misuk. *Hanguk kŭndaesŏng, kŭ kiwŏn ŭl ch'ajasŏ: minjok, seksyu'ŏllit'i, pyŏngnihak* [Finding the origin of Korea's modernity: Race, sexuality, pathology]. Seoul: Ch'ek sesang, 2001.

Koven, Seth, and Sonya Michel. "Womanly Duties: Maternalist Politics and the Origins of the Welfare States in France, Germany, Great Britain, and the United States, 1880–1920." *American Historical Review* 95, no. 4 (1990): 1076–1108.

Koyama Shizuko. *Ryōsai Kenbo: The Educational Ideal of "Good Wife, Wise Mother" in Modern Japan,* translated by Stephen Filler. Leiden, The Netherlands: Brill, 2013.

Kyŏnggi yŏgo 100 nyŏnsa [One hundred years of Kyŏnggi Girls' High School]. Seoul: Kyŏngunhoe, 2009.

Leavitt, Judith. *Brought to Bed: Childbearing in America, 1750–1950.* New York and Oxford: Oxford University Press, 1986.

Lee, Ji-Eun. *Women Pre-Scripted: Forging Modern Roles through Korean Print.* Honolulu: University of Hawai'i Press, 2015.

Liu, Lydia. *Translingual Practice: Literature, National Culture, and Translated Modernity—China, 1900–1937.* Redwood City, CA: Stanford University Press, 1995.

Liu, Michael Shiying. *Prescribing Colonialization: The Role of Medical Practices and Policies in Japan-Ruled Taiwan, 1895–1945.* Ann Arbor, MI: Association for Asian Studies, 2009.

Lo, Ming-cheng M. *Doctors within Borders: Profession, Ethnicity, and Modernity in Colonial Taiwan.* Berkeley and Los Angeles: University of California Press, 2002.

Meckel, Richard A. *Save the Babies: American Public Health Reform and the Prevention of Infant Mortality, 1850–1920.* Baltimore: Johns Hopkins University Press, 1990.

Miki Sakae. *Chōsen igakkushi oyobi shippeishi* [History of Korean medicine and of disease in Korea]. Osaka, Japan: Shibun chuppansha, 1963.

Nihon isekiroku, furoku, igaku hakushi roku, hōki [Japanese medical directory: Appendix, index of medical doctorate (PhD), laws and regulation]. Tokyo: Iji jironsi zōhan, 1926.

No Pyŏnghŭi. *Yŏja sohak susinsŏ.* Reprinted in Hangukhak munhŏn yŏnguso, ed., *Hanguk kaehwagi kyogwasŏ ch'ongsŏ* [Collection of textbooks from the *kaehwa* period], vol. 10, 535–614. Seoul: Asea munhwasa, 1977.

Nolte, Sharon, and Sally Ann Hastings. "The Meiji State's Policy Toward Women, 1890–1910." In *Recreating Japanese Women, 1600–1945,* edited by Gail Lee Bernstein, 151–174. Berkeley and Los Angeles: University of California Press, 1991.

Norgren, Tiana. *Abortion Before Birth Control: The Politics of Reproduction in Postwar Japan.* Princeton, NJ: Princeton University Press, 2001.

O Sŏngch'ŏl. *Singminji ch'odŭng kyoyuk ŭi hyŏngsŏng* [Formation of elementary education in the colonial period]. Seoul: Kyoyuk kwahaksa, 2000.

———, ed. *Singminji kyoyuk yongu ŭi tabyŏnhwa* [Diversification of studies on colonial period education]. P'aju, South Korea: Kyoyuk kwahaksa, 2011.

Oak, Sung-Deuk, ed. *Sources of Korean Christianity, 1832–1945.* Seoul: The Institute for Korean Church History, 2004.

Oh, Se-mi. "Letters to the Editor: Women, Newspapers, and the Public Sphere in Turn-of-the Century Korea." In *Epistolary Letters: Letters in the Communicative Space of the Chosŏn, 1392–1910,* edited by Ja-Hyun Kim Haboush, 162–167. New York: Columbia University Press, 2009.

Otsubo, Sumiko. "The Female Body and Eugenic Thought in Meiji Japan." In *Building a Modern Japan: Science, Technology, and Medicine in the Meiji Era and Beyond,* edited by Morris Low, 61–81. New York: Palgrave MacMillan, 2005.

Paek Okkyŏng. "Chosŏn sidae ch'ulsan e taehan insik kwa silje" [A study on the thought and historical fact about birth during the Chosŏn dynasty]. *Ewha sahak yŏngu* 34 (2007): 191–207.

Pak Chŏngdong. *Ch'odŭng susin* [Elementary morals] (1909). Reprinted in *Hanguk kaehwagi kyogwasŏ ch'ongsŏ* 9. Seoul: Asea munhwasa, 1977.

———, trans. *Sinch'an kajŏnghak.* Seoul: Chŏnghŭijin, 1907.

Pak Chongsŏk. *Kaehwagi Hanguk ŭi kwahak kyogwasŏ* [Science textbooks of Korea during the Enlightenment period]. Seoul: Hanguk haksul chŏngbo, 2007.

———. "Kaehwagi kwahak kyoyukcha ŭi paegyŏng kwa yŏkhwal [Background and role of science educators of the Kaehwa period]." *Hanguk kwahak kyoyukhak hoeji,* 20, no. 3 (2000): 443–454.

Pak Myŏnggyu and Sŏ Hoch'ul. *Singmin kwŏllyŏk kwa t'onggye: Chosŏn ch'ongdokpu ŭi t'onggye wa sensŏsŭ* [Colonial authority and statistics: Statistics and census of the GGK]. Seoul: Seoul National University Press, 2003.

Pak Pyŏnggi and Kim Minjae. *Kŭndae hakpu p'yŏnch'an susinsŏ* [Susin textbooks published by the modern board of education]. Seoul: Somyŏng, 2012.

Pak Sŏnmi. "Chosŏn sidae ŭinyŏ koyuk yŏngu, kŭ yangsŏng kwa hwaldong ŭl chungsimŭro" [A study of education of *ŭinyŏ* during the Chosŏn period, their development and activity]. PhD diss., Chungang Univeristy, 1994.

———. *Kŭndae yŏsŏng, cheguk ŭl kŏch'ŏ Chosŏn ŭro hoeyuhada, singminji munhwa chibae wa Ilbon yuhak.* P'aju, South Korea: Ch'angbi, 2007. Originally published in Japan by Yamakawa Shuppansha, 2003.

Pak Yongok. "1905–1910 nyŏn sŏgu kŭndae yŏsŏngsang e taehan ihae wa insik" [Understanding of Western modern womanhood, 1905–1910." In *Hanguk yŏsŏng kŭndaehwa ŭi yŏksachŏk maengnak*, 297–339. Seoul: Chisik sanŏpsa, 2001.

Pak Yunjae (Park Yun-jae). "1876–1904 nyŏn Ilbon kwannip pyŏngwŏn ŭi sŏllip kwa hwaltong e kwanhan yŏngu" [A study on the establishment and activity of Japanese government hospitals in Korea, 1876–1904]. *Yŏksa wa hyŏnsil* 42 (2001): 179–206.

———. "The 1927 Emetine Injection Incident in Colonial Korea and the Intervention Emetine incident." *Korea Journal* 50, no. 1 (2010): 160–177.

———. "1930~1940 nyŏndae Cho Hŏnyŏng ŭi hanŭihak insik kwa tongsŏ chŏlch'ungchŏk ŭihangnon" [Jo Heonyeong's understanding of and vision for the future of Korean traditional medicine in the 1930–1940s]. *Hanguk kŭnhyŏndaesa yŏngu* 40 (2007): 118–139, 260–261.

———. *Hanguk kŭndae ŭihak ŭi kiwŏn* [The origin of the Korean modern medical system]. Seoul: Hyean, 2005.

———. "Ilcheha ŭisa kyech'ŭng ŭi sŏngjang kwa chŏngch'esŏng hyŏngsŏng" [The growth of physicians and formation of their subjectivity under Japanese colonial rule]. *Yŏksa wa hyŏnsil* 63 (2007): 163–189.

———. "Taehan chegukki chongdu ŭi yangŏngso ŭi sŏllip kwa hwaltong" [Establishment of the training school for vaccinators and their activities during the Taehan Empire]. *Chŏngsin munhwa yŏngu* 32, no. 4 (2009): 29–54.

———. "Yangsaengesŏ wisaenguro, kaehwap'a ŭi ŭihangnon kwa kŭndae kukka kŏnsŏl" [From *yangsaeng* to *wisaeng*, medical discourse of the Kaehwa group and construction of the modern state]. *Sahoe wa yŏksa* 63 (2003): 30–50.

Park, Jin-kyung. "Bodies for Empire: Biopolitics, Reproduction, and Sexual Knowledge in Late Colonial Korea." *Ŭisahak* 23, no. 2 (2014): 203–238.

———. "Corporeal Colonialism: Medicine, Reproduction, and Race in Colonial Korea." PhD diss., University of Illinois, Urbana-Champaign, 2008.

———. "Husband Murder as the 'Sickness' of Korea: Carceral Gynecology, Race, and Tradition in Colonial Korea, 1926–1932." *Journal of Women's History* 25, no. 3 (2013): 116–140.

———. "Interrogating the 'Population Problem' of the Non-Western Empire: Japanese Colonialism, the Korean Peninsula, and the Global Geopolitics of Race." *Interventions: International Journal of Postcolonial Studies* 19, no. 8 (2017): 1112–1131.

———. "Managing 'Dis-ease': Print Media, Medical Images, and Patent Medicine Advertisements in Colonial Korea." *International Journal of Cultural Studies*. First published January 13, 2017.

———. "Picturing Empire and Illness: Biomedicine, Venereal Disease, and the Modern Girl in Korea under Japanese Colonial Rule." *Cultural Studies* 28, no. 1 (2014): 108–141.

———. "Yellow Men's Burden: East Asian Imperialism, Forensic Medicine, and Conjugality in Colonial Korea." *Acta Koreana* 18, no. 1 (2015): 187–207.

Park, Seong Rae. *Science and Technology in Korean History: Excursions, Innovations, and Issues.* Fremont, CA: Jain Publishing Company, 2005.

Pettid, Michael J. "Confucian Educational Works for Upper Status Women in Chosŏn." In *Women and Confucianism in Chosŏn Korea*, edited by Michael J. Pettid and Youngmin Kim, 49–70. Albany: State University of New York Press, 2011.

Pinghŏgak Yi ssi. *Kyuhap ch'ongsŏ.* Translated by Yi Minsu. Seoul: Kirinwŏn, 1988.

Porter, Dorothy. *Health Citizenship: Essays in Social Medicine and Biomedical Politics.* Berkeley and Los Angeles: University of California Press, 2011.

Robinson, Michael. *Cultural Nationalism in Colonial Korea, 1920–1925.* Seattle: University of Washington Press, 1988.

Rogaski, Ruth. *Hygienic Modernity: Meanings of Health and Disease in Treaty-Port China.* Berkeley and Los Angeles: University of California Press, 2004.

Rousseau, Julie. "Enduring Labors: The 'New Midwife'; and the Modern Culture of Childbearing in Early 20th Century Japan." PhD diss., Columbia University, 1998.

Sand, Jordan. *House and Home in Modern Japan: Architecture, Domestic Space, and Bourgeois Culture, 1880–1930.* Cambridge, MA: Harvard University Press, 2004.

Sauer, Charles A. *Within the Gate.* Seoul: Korea Methodist News Service, 1934.

Schmid, Andre. *Korea Between Empires, 1895–1919.* New York: Columbia University Press, 2002.

Sharrocks, A. M. *T'aemo wisaeng* [The hygiene of parturition]. Seoul: Methodist Publishing House, 1905.

Shemo, Connie. *The Chinese Medical Ministries of Kang Cheng and Shi Meiyu, 1872–1937: On a Cross-Cultural Frontier of Gender, Race, and Nation.* Bethlehem, PA: Lehigh University Press, 2011.

Shin In Sup and Shin Kie Hyuk. *Advertising in Korea.* Seoul: Communication Books Publications, 2004.

Shorter, Edward. *Women's Bodies: A Social History of Women's Encounter with Health, Ill-health, and Medicine,* 2nd ed. New Brunswick, NJ, and London: Transaction Publishers, 1991.

Sin Ch'anggŏn. "Cho Hŏnyŏng ŭi chŏngch'ijŏk ŭihak sasang—singminjigi, haebang hu, 'nanbuk' hu rŭl t'onghayŏ," [Cho Heon-Yeong's political thought of medicine]. *Hang'uksa ron* 42:115–151.

Sin Kyuhwan and Sŏ Honggwan. "Hanguk kŭndae sarip pyŏngwŏn ŭi paljŏn kwajŏng, 1885 nyŏn-1960 nyŏn kkaji" [The development of private hospitals in modern Korea, 1885–1960]. *Ŭisahak* 11, no. 1 (2002): 85–110.

Sin Tongun. "Hyongbŏp kaejŏng kwa kwallyŏn pon nakt'aejoe yŏngu" [A study of abortion from the viewpoint of criminal law reform in Korea]. *Hyŏngsa chŏngch'aek yŏngu* [Study of criminal policy] 2, no. 2 (1991): 333–381.

Sin Tongwŏn (Shin Dong-won). "Chosŏn hugi ŭiyak saenghwal ŭi pyŏnhwa: sŏnmul kyŏngje esŏ sijang kyŏngje ro, 'Miam ilgi,' 'Soe mirok,' 'Yichae nango,' 'Hŭmyŏng' ŭi punsok" [Shift in everyday medical practices; from gift economy to market economy]. *Yŏksa pip'yŏng* 75 (2006): 353.

———. *Hanguk kŭndae pogŏn ŭiryosa* [History of health and medicine in modern Korea]. Seoul: Hanul Academy, 1997.

———. *Hoyŏlja Chosŏnŭl sŭpkyŏkhada: mom kwa ŭihak ŭi Hanguksa* [Cholera invades Chosŏn: History of the body and medicine in Korea]. Seoul: Yŏksa pip'yŏngsa, 2004.

———. "Ilche ŭi pogŏn ŭiryo chŏngch'aek mit Hangugin ŭi kŏngang sangt'ae e kwanhan yŏngu" [A study on the policy of health services and Koreans' health state in Japanese colonial state]. MA thesis, Seoul National University, 1986.

———. "Pyŏn'gang soegaro ingnŭn sŏng, pyŏng, chugŏm ŭi munhwasa" [Reading *Pyŏn'gang soegaro*, a cultural history of sexuality, disease, and death]. *Yŏksa pip'yŏng* 67 (2004): 307–332.

———. "Western Medicine, Korean Government, and Imperialism in Late Nineteenth-Century Korea: The Cases of the Chosŏn Government Hospital and Smallpox Vaccination." *Historia Scientiarum* 13, no. 3 (2004): 164–175.

Sin Tongwŏn, Kim Nam'il, and Yŏ Insŏk. *Hangwŏnŭro ingnŭn* Tongŭi pogam [Reading the *Tongŭi pogam* in one volume]. Seoul: Tŭllyŏk, 1999.

Sin Yongha. "Uri nara ch'oech'o ŭi kŭndae hakkyo sŏllip e taehayŏ" [On the establishment of the first modern school in Korea]. *Hanguksa yŏngu* 10, no. 9 (1974): 191–204.

Sin Yŏngjŏn. "Singminji Chosŏn esŏ usaeng undong ŭi chŏngae wa sŏnggyŏk: 1930 nyŏndae 'Usaeng' ŭl chungsimŭro" [The characteristics of Korea's eugenic movement in the colonial period represented in the bulletin *Usaeng*]. *Ŭisahak* 15, no. 2 (2006): 133–155.

Smith-Rosenberg, Carroll, and Charles Rosenberg. "The Female Animal: Medical and Biological Views of Woman and Her Role in Nineteenth-Century America." *Journal of American History* 60 (1973): 332–356.

So Hyŏnsuk. "Ilche sigi ch'ulsan chehan tamnon yŏngu" [Study of the birth control discourse in colonial Korea]. *Yŏksa wa hyŏnsil* [History and reality] 38 (Winter 2000): 221–253.

———. "'Kŭndae' e ŭi yŏlmang kwa ilsang saenghwal ŭi singminhwa: Ilche sigi saenghwal kaesŏn undong kwa jendŏ chŏngch'i rŭl chungsimŭro" [Desire for the "modern" and colonization of everyday life: Lifestyle improvement campaign and gender politics during Japanese colonial rule]. In *Ilsangsa ro ponŭn Hanguk kŭnhyŏndaesa: Hanguk kwa Togil ilsangsa ŭi saeroun mannam* [Korean modern history through history of the everyday: The meeting of Korean and German history], edited by Yi Sangnok and Yi Yunjae, 119–173. Seoul: Ch'aek kwa hamkke, 2006.

Solinger, Rickie. *Reproductive Politics: What Everyone Needs to Know.* New York: Oxford University Press, 2013.

Song Insu. *Hanguk yŏsŏng kyoyuksa* [History of Korean women's education]. Seoul: Yonsei University Press, 1977.

Stage, Sarah, and Virginia B. Vincenti, eds. *Rethinking Home Economics: Women and the History of a Profession.* Ithaca, NY, and London: Cornell University Press, 1997.

Suh, So Young. "Korean Medicine Between the Local and the Universal: 1600–1945." PhD diss., University of California, Los Angeles, 2006.

Suh, Soyoung. *Naming the Local: Medicine, Language, and Identity in Korea since the Fifteenth Century.* Cambridge, MA: Harvard University Asia Center, 2017.

Tatsumi, Yukako. "Constructing Home Economics in Imperial Japan." PhD diss., University of Maryland, College Park, 2011.

Terazawa, Yuki. "Gender, Knowledge, and Power: Reproductive Medicine in Japan, 1790–1930." PhD diss., University of California, Los Angeles, 2001.

Tikhonov, Vladimir. "Masculinizing the Nation: Gender Ideologies in Traditional Korea and in the 1890s–1900s Korean Enlightenment Discourse." *Journal of Asian Studies* 66, no. 4 (2007): 1029–1065.

Underwood, Lillias H. *Fifteen Years Among the Top-Knots.* Boston, New York, and Chicago: American Tract Society, 1904. Reprint. Seoul: Kyung-in Publishing, Co., 1977.

United Presbyterian Church in the U.S.A. Commission on Ecumenical Mission and Relations, Secretaries' Files: Korea Mission, 1903–1972, RG 140. Presbyterian Historical Society, Philadelphia, Pennsylvania.

Wells, J. H. *Wisaeng* [Introduction to hygiene], 2nd ed. Seoul: Korean Religious Tract Society, 1907.

Woman's Foreign Missionary Society, Methodist Episcopal Church. *Annual Reports of the Korea Woman's Conference* [*KWC*], 1898–1931.

Wood, Ann Douglas. "'The Fashionable Diseases': Women's Complaints and Their Treatment in Nineteenth-Century America." *The Journal of Interdisciplinary History* 4 (1973): 25–52.

Wu, Yili. *Reproducing Women: Medicine, Metaphor, and Childbirth in Late Imperial China.* Berkeley and Los Angeles: University of California Press, 2010.

Yang Hyŏna. "Hoju chedo: Hanguk ŭi singminjisŏnggwa kabujangje ŭi ch'ukto" [The family-headship system: The epitome of Korean coloniality and patriarchy]. In *Kyŏnggye ŭi yŏsngtŭl: Hanguk kŭndae yŏsŏngsa* [Women on the border: History of women in modern Korea], edited by Seoul National University Institute for Gender Research [*Yŏsŏng yŏnguso*], 40–78. Seoul: Hanul Academy, 2013.

Yi Chiyŏn and Chŏn Sangsuk. "Singminji sigi kŭndaejŏk whisikŭrosŏ kajŏnghak ŭi hyŏngsŏng" [Formation of home economics as modern scientific knowledge during the colonial period in Korea]. *Ewha sahak yŏngu* [Studies of Ewha history] 52 (2016): 69–97.

———. "Singminji sigi yŏsŏng kodŭng kyoyuk kwa kajŏnghak ŭi chedohwa" [The systematization of women's high school education and home economics during the colonial period in Korea]. *Chiyŏk kwa yŏksa* 36 (2015): 247–280.

Yi Ch'ungho. *Hanguk ŭisa kyoyuksa yŏngu* [History of the education of physicians in Korea]. Seoul: Hanguk charyowŏn, 1998.

Yi Kkonme (Yi Ggod Me). "Han Singwang: *Hanguk* kŭndae ŭi sanp'a ija kanhoburosŏ ŭi sam" [Han Singwang: Her life as a modern midwife and nurse]. *Ŭisahak* 15, no. 1 (2006): 107–119.

———. "Hanguk chiyŏk sahoe kanho ŭi sŏguja Yi Kŭmjŏn e kwanhan yŏksachŏk koch'al" [Historical review of Lee Keumjeon, a pioneer in community health nursing in Korea]. *Chiyŏk sahoe kanhohak hoeji* 24, no. 1 (2013): 74–86.

———. *Hanguk kŭndae kanhosa* [History of modern nursing in Korea]. Seoul: Hanul Academy, 2002.

———. "Hanguk ŭi udubŏp to'ip kwa silsi e kwanhan yŏngu: 1876 nyŏn esŏ 1910 nyŏn kkajirŭl chungsimŭro" [A study of the entrance and assimilation of cowpox vaccination in Korea, with a focus on the years between 1876 and 1910]. MA thesis, Seoul National University, 1992.

———. "Ilbanin ŭi hanŭihak insik kwa ŭiyak iyong" [A study on the general public understanding and utilization of traditional Korean medicine in the colonial period]. In *Hanŭihak, singminji rŭl alt'a: singminji sigi hanŭihak ŭi kŭndaehwa yŏngu* [The modernization of Korean traditional medicine during the colonial period], edited by Yŏnse taehakkyo ŭihaksa yŏnguso [Institute for History of Medicine, Yonsei University]. 137–154. Seoul: Ak'anet, 2008.

———. "Ilche kangjŏmgi sanp'a Chŏng Chongmyŏng sam kwa taejung undong" [Life and activism of Chŏng Chongmyŏng, a midwife during the colonial period]. *Ŭisahak* 21, no. 3 (2012): 551–592.

———. "Ilche sidae ŭi ti kanho tanch'e e kwanhan koch'al: Chosŏn kanhobuhoe ŭi sujun hyangsang noryŏk kwa Chosŏn kanhobu hyŏphoe ŭi sahoe hwaltong" [Study of nursing associations during Japanese colonial rule: The effort to elevate status of Korean Nurses' Association and social activities of the Korean Nurses' Society]. *Kanho haengjŏnghak hoeji* 6, no. 3 (2000): 421–429.

Yi Kkonme and Hwang Sangik. "Uri nara kŭndae pyŏngwŏn esŏ ŭi kanho" [Nursing in Korea's modern hospitals]. *Ŭisahak* 6, no. 1 (1997): 55–72.

Yi Mungŏn. *Yangarok* [Records of raising a child], translated by Yi Sangju. Seoul: T'aehaksa, 1997.

Yi Myŏnu. "Kŭndae kyoyukki (1876–1910) hakhoejirŭl t'onghan kwahak kyuyuk ŭi chŏngae" [Science education through journals of academic societies 1876–1910]. *Journal of Korean Earth Science Society* 22, no. 3 (2001): 75–88.

Yi Pangwŏn. "Pak Esther (1877–1910) ŭi saengae wa ŭiryo sŏngyo hwaltong" [Life and medical activities of Esther Pak (1877–1910)]. *Ŭisahak* 16, no. 2 (2007): 193–213.

———. "Pogunyŏngwan ŭi sŏllip kwa hwaltong" [The establishment and activities of Pogunyŏgwan]. *Ŭisahak* 17, no. 1 (2008): 37–56.

Yi Sugin. "'Kajŏng' (家政) ŭl t'onghae pon 18 segi ŭi saenghwal segye" [Eighteenth-century everyday life as seen through *Kajŏng*]. *Hanguk munhwa* 51 (2010): 65–88.

Yi Tŏkchu. *T'aehwa kidokkyo sahoe pokchigwan ŭi yŏksa: 1921–1993* [History of Taihwa Christian Community Center]. Seoul: T'aehwa kidokkyo sahoe pokchigwan, 1993.

Yŏ Insŏk, Pak Yunjae, Yi Kyŏngnok, and Pak Hyŏngu. "Hanguk ŭisa myŏnhŏ chedo ŭi chŏngch'ak kwajŏng—Hanmal kwa Ilche sidaerŭl chungsimŭro" [A history of the medical licensing system in Korea from the Taehan to the Japanese colonial period]. *Ŭisahak* 11, no. 2 (2002): 137–153.

Yŏ Insŏk and Yi Kyuch'ang. "Hansŏng ŭisahoe e taehayŏ" [On Hansung Physicians' Association]. *Ŭisahak* 1, no. 1 (1992): 31–35.

Yŏnse taehakkyo ŭihaksa yŏnguso [Institute for History of Medicine, Yonsei University], ed. "Chosansa int'ŏbu chŏngni" [Overview of interviews with midwives]. *Yŏnse ŭisahak* [Yonsei Journal of Medical History] 11, no. 2 (2008): 87–91.

———. *Hanŭihak, singminji rŭl alta: singminji sigi hanŭihak ŭi kŭndaehwa yŏngu* [The modernization of Korean traditional medicine during the colonial period]. Seoul: Ak'anet, 2008.

———. "Samil pyŏngwŏn sŏllipja, Yu Sŭnghŏn" [Founder of Samil Hospital, Yi Sŭnghŏn]. *Yŏnse ŭisahak* 12, no. 2 (2009): 59–103.

Yoo, Theodore Jun. *It's Madness: The Politics of Mental Health in Colonial Korea.* Oakland: University of California Press, 2016.

———. "The 'New Woman' and the Politics of Love, Marriage and Divorce in Colonial Korea." *Gender & History* 17, no. 2 (2005): 295–324.

———. *The Politics of Gender in Colonial Korea: Education, Labor, and Health, 1910–1945.* Berkeley and Los Angeles: University of California Press, 2008.

Yu Kilchun. "Observations on a Journey to the West." Edited by John B. Duncan and translated by Hanmee Na Kim et al. Unpublished manuscript, last modified January 25, 2017. Microsoft Word file.

———. *Sŏyu kyŏnmun*, translated by Hŏ Kyŏngjin. Seoul: Sŏhae munjip, 2004.

Yuh, Leighanne Kimberly. "Education, the Struggle for Power, and Identity Formation in Korea, 1876–1910." PhD diss., University of California, Los Angeles, 2008.

———. "Guns, Farms, and Foreign Languages: The Introduction of Western Learning and the First Government Schools in Late Nineteenth-Century Korea." *Paedagogica Historica* 52, no. 6 (2016): 580–595.

———. "Moral Education, Modernization Imperatives, and the *People's Elementary Reader* (1895): Accommodation in the Early History of Modern Education in Korea." *Acta Koreana* 18, no. 2 (2015): 327–355.

INDEX

Page numbers in boldface type refer to tables.

abortion: birth control and, 109, 125, 127, 139; comfort women and, 201n13; New Midwife and, 86, 181n46; regulation of, 125–126, 137
acupuncture, 4, 54, 116, 118, 142n13, 168n23
Allen, Horace, 5, 7, 51, 52, 54, 141n7
Avison, Douglas, 99, 169n27, 187n117
Avison, Oliver R., 63, 169n27

biomedicine, 6–8, 55, 170n43; *hanbang* and, 116–117, 192n36; physicians of, 56–57, 110, 161n99, 167n8
birth control (*sana chehan/chojŏl*): conflation with abortion, 125, 197n82; contraceptives, 126, 197n90, 198n100; eugenics and, 129–130, 137, 183n70, 199n104; Ishimoto Shizue, 136, 200n9; opposition to, 199n103, regulation of, 126, 136, 139; reproductive health and, 10, 12, 126; rhythm method, 127, 197n90, 198n91; Seoul Youth Association debate, 108–109; woman-centered positions on, 127–129, 132. *See also* population; sex education
Bording, Maren, 99, 104–105
Burns, Susan, 122

cancer, 115, 131, 190n12, 191n21
Chang Ch'ŏnyŏng, 127
Chang Mungyŏng, 72, 194n49
Ch'anyanghoe (Promotion Society), 2, 17, 28, 33, 141n4, 148n6
charity hospital (*chahye ŭiwŏn*): medical missionaries and, 91–92; midwifery training, 85, 90; Sorokdo, 171n44; system, 7–8, 47, 59, 145n30, 170nn42, 43
Chasŏn puinhoe chapchi, 40
Chejungwŏn, 5, 7, 51, 59, 81, 141n7, 144n20. *See also* Severance Hospital
childbearing complications, 89, 119–121; fistula, 113, 119, 120, 121; maternal mortality, 121, 133; prolapsed uterus, 114, 119, 120. *See also* maternal health; *puinbyŏng*
childbirth: in Chosŏn, 20, 86, 181n47; dangers of, 119–121; delaying and spacing, 129, 131; medicalized, 9; postpartum care, 20, 114, 121; prenatal care, 45–46, 98, 100, 105, 131, 136, 139, 151n19; standardizing, 9, 89; in the West, 86, 194n56. *See also* obstetrics
child-rearing: in Chosŏn, 20–21; Domestic Sciences and, 40, 44–47, 96, 110, 165n131, 165n134; as gendered practice, 14, 31, 109, 126, 127, 137, 139; medicalization of, 50, 100, 107

ABOUT THE AUTHOR

Sonja M. Kim is associate professor in the Department of Asian and Asian American Studies at Binghamton University, the State University of New York.

HAWAI‘I STUDIES ON KOREA

WAYNE PATTERSON
The Ilse: First-Generation Korean Immigrants, 1903–1973

LINDA S. LEWIS
Laying Claim to the Memory of May: A Look Back at the 1980
Kwangju Uprising

MICHAEL FINCH
Min Yŏng-gwan: A Political Biography

MICHAEL J. SETH
Education Fever: Society, Politics, and the Pursuit of Schooling in
South Korea

CHAN E. PARK
Voices from the Straw Mat: Toward an Ethnography of Korean
Story Singing

ANDREI N. LANKOV
Crisis in North Korea: The Failure of De-Stalinization, 1956

HAHN MOON-SUK
And So Flows History

TIMOTHY R. TANGHERLINI AND SALLIE YEA, EDITORS
Sitings: Critical Approaches to Korean Geography

ALEXANDER VOVIN
Koreo-Japonica: A Re-evaluation of a Common Genetic Origin

YUNG-HEE KIM
Questioning Minds: Short Stories of Modern Korean Women
Writers

TATIANA GABROUSSENKO
Soldiers on the Cultural Front: Developments in the Early History
of North Korean Literature and Literary Policy

KYUNG-AE PARK, EDITOR
Non-Traditional Security Issues in North Korea

CHARLOTTE HORLYCK AND MICHAEL J. PETTID, EDITORS
Death, Mourning, and the Afterlife in Korea: Critical Aspects of
Death from Ancient to Contemporary Times

CARL F. YOUNG
Eastern Learning and the Heavenly Way: The Tonghak and
Ch'ŏndogyo Movements and the Twilight of Korean Independence

DON BAKER, WITH FRANKLIN RAUSCH
Catholics and Anti-Catholicism in Chosŏn Korea

SONJA M. KIM
Imperatives of Care: Women and Medicine in Colonial Korea